Atlas of

BULLOUS DISEASES

Atlas of
BULLOUS DISEASES

Lionel Fry BSc MD FRCP

Emeritus Professor of Dermatology
Imperial College
London, UK

informa
healthcare

First published in the United Kingdom in 2006 by Informa Healthcare, 4 Park Square, Milton Park, Abingdon, Oxon OX14 4RN. Informa Healthcare is a trading division of Informa UK Ltd. Registered Office: 37/41 Mortimer Street, London W1T 3JH. Registered in England and Wales Number 1072954.

Tel.: +44 (0)20 7017 6000
Fax: +44 (0)20 7017 6699
E-mail: info.medicine@tandf.co.uk
Website: www.informahealthcare.com

A CIP record for this book is available from the British Library.

Library of Congress Cataloging-in-Publication Data

Data available on application

ISBN10: 0-415-38338-2
ISBN13: 978-0-415-38338-7

Distributed in North and South America by

Taylor & Francis
6000 Broken Sound Parkway, NW, (Suite 300)
Boca Raton, FL 33487, USA

Within Continental USA
Tel.: 1(800)272 7737; Fax: 1(800)374 3401
Outside Continental USA
Tel.: (561)994 0555; Fax: (561)361 6018
E-mail: orders@crcpress.com

Distributed in the rest of the world by
Thomson Publishing Services
Cheriton House
North Way
Andover, Hampshire SP10 5BE, UK
Tel.: +44 (0)1264 332424
E-mail: tps.tandfsalesorder@thomson.com

Composition by Parthenon Publishing

Printed and bound by T.G. Hostench S.A., Spain

Contents

Preface

The bullous or blistering diseases is an arbitrary term because many of the common skin disorders, e.g. eczema, erythema multiforme, impetigo, drug eruptions, and insect bites may also have blisters in their clinical presentation but are not included under this heading.

The term bullous disorders dates from the latter half of the nineteenth century and was used to refer to dermatitis herpetiformis, pemphigoid, and pemphigus. The name 'bullous diseases' has remained and other disorders similar to the original three are now included. This extended group of disorders is now often referred to as the 'immunobullous diseases' because immunological mechanisms are involved. However, the term 'autoimmune bullous diseases' is sometimes used because they are considered to be autoimmune.

The concept of autoimmunity, however, is now being questioned as it is thought that the so-called autoimmune diseases may be precipitated and even maintained, by micro-organisms. The future will decide the terminology of this group of diseases.

The main reason for agreeing to write this book has been my interest in dermatitis herpetiformis over the last forty years. This is a fascinating disease, which has been shown to be gluten dependent. Immunological mechanisms are involved in the pathogenesis and autoantibodies occur but this is a disease due to, and maintained by, an external antigen.

The book will hopefully prove to be of interest to dermatologists, immunologists and pathologists. There is still a great deal of further work to be done before the exact causes and pathogenetic mechanisms are finally elucidated.

I gratefully acknowledge the illustrations provided by Professor Fenella Wojnarowska and Dr Nick Francis. My thanks also to Mrs Fiona Smith for help with the manuscript.

Lionel Fry
Imperial College
London, 2006

1 Introduction and history

INTRODUCTION

The so-called 'bullous eruptions' comprise a group of skin disorders in which one of the main features is a bulla or blister. Essentially this is a raised lesion filled with tissue fluid and may be small, < 5 mm, and sometimes referred to as a vesicle, or large, > 5 mm and sometimes up to 3 cm, and sometimes referred to as a bulla. The definition of the bullous disorders is somewhat arbitrary, because many other skin disorders which are definite entities may also exhibit blisters as one of the features of their presentation, e.g. insect bites, erythema multiforme, impetigo, fungal and viral infections and eczema. The skin diseases grouped under the term 'bullous' are considered to have an autoimmune basis, with demonstrable antibodies directed against specific components of the skin. Excluded from this group of disorders is epidermolysis bullosa. The clinical types of this disease are due to specific gene defects, and are usually considered to be distinct entities and not one of the so-called bullous disorders.

HISTORY

The three diseases grouped as 'bullous' in the latter half of the 19th century were dermatitis herpetiformis (DH), pemphigus and pemphigoid, and were not distinguished from each other. In 1884 an American dermatologist, Duhring, described DH as a protean entity and mentioned six types depending on the predominant clinical lesion: erythematous, vesiculosa, bullosa, pustulosa, papulosa and multiformis. At the time, many dermatologists did not agree with Duhring and found difficulty in distinguishing DH from other bullous disorders. In fact Kaposi (1891) described Duhring's concept as a diagnosis of confusion. However, Duhring was supported by Brocq (1898), who emphasized that the skin lesions in DH were indeed frequently polymorphic and not simply 'blisters'.

It was nearly 50 years later before any other significant contribution was made, when Civatte (1943) described acantholysis (separation of the epidermal cells from each other) in the blisters of pemphigus and loss of intercellular bridges between the epidermal cells in the surrounding skin. These findings enabled pemphigus to be distinguished by histological features from other disorders presenting with blisters. The term pemphigoid was introduced by Lever in 1953 to distinguish patients who were thought to have pemphigus but had a subepidermal blister on microscopy. However, there was still confusion over the classification of disorders found with subepidermal blisters on histology. Not only was it too difficult to distinguish between pemphigoid and dermatitis herpetiformis, erythema multiforme also had subepidermal blisters on light microscopy. The distinction between DH and pemphigoid was made possible in the 1950s, following the observation that dapsone was effective in clearing the rash of DH and that it relapsed when the drug was discontinued. The problem with this criterion was that other skin disorders also improved with dapsone, e.g. vasculitis, subcorneal pustular dermatosis, linear immunoglobulin A (IgA) disease, some patients with pemphigus and some with eczema.

The most definitive diagnostic criteria were established in the 1960s and 1970s based on direct and indirect immunofluorescent tests. In the 1960s, circulating IgG antibodies were found that bound to the basement membrane zone in pemphigoid and the intercellular region in the epidermis in pemphigus. When direct immunofluorescence is used as the diagnostic test it is important to take specimens from the perilesional skin, because in lesional skin the immunoglobulins may be destroyed by enzymes produced in the inflammatory reaction.

In the 1970s, IgA deposits were found in the dermal papillae and occasionally in a linear pattern below the basement membrane in DH. The presence of IgA in the uninvolved skin is now the diagnostic criterion for DH. In the 1970s it was also found that some patients who had a bullous eruption which responded to dapsone as well as IgA in the uninvolved skin were different from DH patients. This group had a different distribution of their eruption, they did not have associated gluten-sensitive enteropathy and the IgA deposition was homogeneous along the line of the basement membrane. This group of patients were termed 'linear IgA disease', and this is now recognized as a distinct entity. It is most important to distinguish between a linear homogeneous pattern of IgA deposition along the line of the basement membrane as in linear IgA disease, and a granular distribution (i.e. with breaks) in the linear IgA deposition which may be seen in DH and has been termed 'linear granular'.

In the 1970s and 1980s, immunoglobulin deposits were also found in the basement membrane region of mucous membrane (cicatricial) pemphigoid, epidermolysis bullosa acquisita and pemphigoid gestationis.

In an attempt to increase the diagnostic significance of the immunoglobulin deposits in those disorders with basement membrane deposition, the split-skin technique was developed in the 1980s. In this technique the biopsy specimen is exposed to 1 mol/l NaCl, which induces a subepidermal blister. In epidermolysis bullosa acquista the immunoglobulins are found on the floor of the blister, and in pemphigoid and pemphigoid gestationis in the roof of the blister (Figures 1.1 and 1.2). In linear IgA disease and mucous membrane pemphigoid the immunoglobulins may be found in the roof or floor of the blister. Using the antibodies found in the bullous disorders has enabled definition of the antigens in the epidermal and basement membrane regions. Thus, it has now been possible to identify the exact sites of immunoglobulin deposition in the skin (Figure 1.3). Determination of the antigens in the bullous disorders in the 1980s and 1990s has helped in their diagnosis.

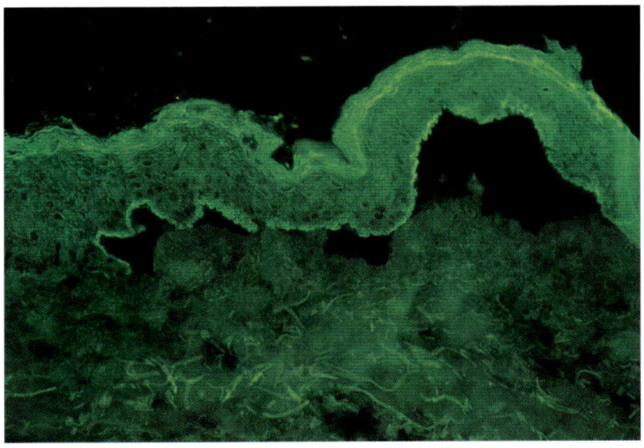

Figure 1.1 Immunoglobulin deposits (IgG) in the roof of the blister in pemphigoid (with kind permission of Professor F. Wojnarowska)

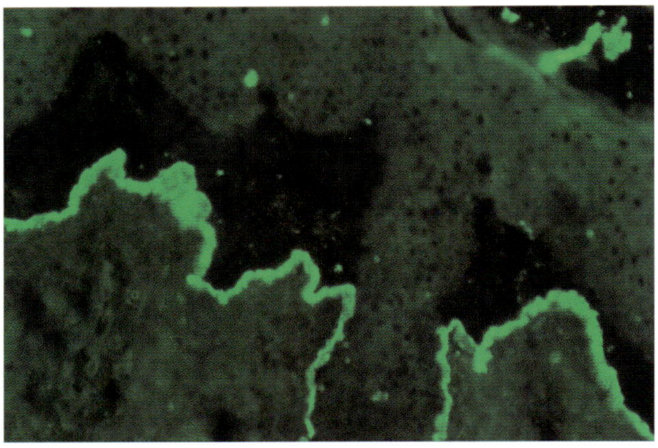

Figure 1.2 Immunoglobulin deposits (IgG) in the floor of the blister in acquired epidermolysis bullosa (with kind permission of Professor F. Wojnarowska)

As with autoimmune disorders in general, the skin disorders in this book are called autoimmune because they have circulating antibodies to known components of the human body. The question that has often been posed is: are these antibodies of a primary nature and pathogenic, or are they secondary to tissue damage and release of neoepitopes to which antibodies develop? In the case of pemphigus and, more recently, pemphigoid, the antibodies have been shown to be pathogenic. However, it is possible that an environmental factor (possibly a micro-organism) may trigger the autoimmune reaction and may even maintain it. Indeed, one of the most significant advances in the understanding of the pathogenesis of

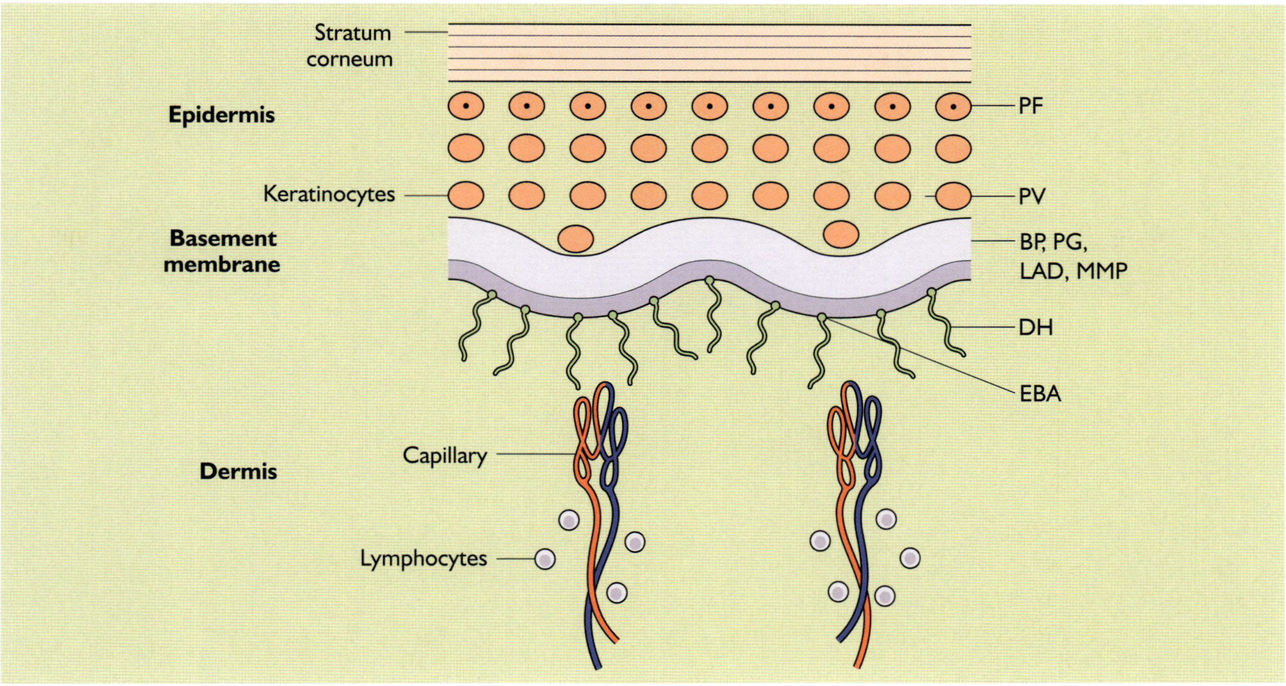

Figure 1.3 Sites of blister formation in bullous disorders. DH, dermatitis herpetiformis; EBA, epidermolysis bullosa acquisita; PF, pemphigus foliaceus; PV, pemphigus vulgaris; BP, bullous pemphigoid; PG, pemphigoid gestationis; LAD, linear IgA disease; MMP, mucous membrane pemphigoid

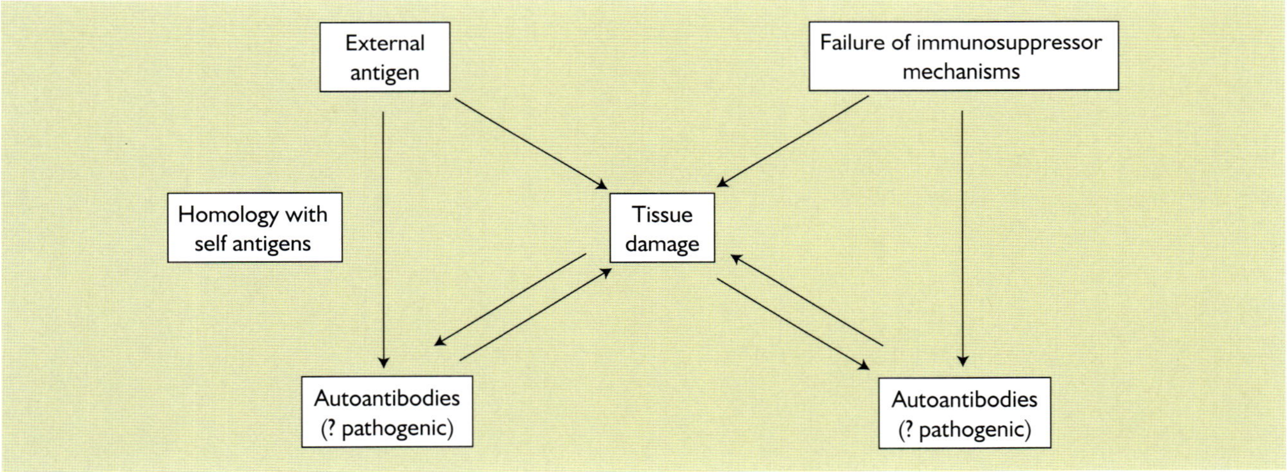

Figure 1.4 Possible pathways in autoimmunity

bullous disorders was the discovery in the late 1960s and 1970s that patients with DH had a gluten-sensitivity enteropathy, identical to that in celiac disease. In addition, the eruption of DH was shown to be gluten-dependent, and avoidance of gluten in the diet results in a 'cure'. Antibodies are found in the serum and may well be pathogenic, i.e. involved in the disease process. However, removal of the external antigen (gluten) results in healing of the pathological end-points of the disease (skin lesions and enteropathy) and disappearance of the antibodies from the circulation.

Thus, in 'so-called' autoimmune diseases the pathological process is initiated by an external agent, the damage to the tissues results in the development of neoepitopes to which antibodies develop and these antibodies can be pathogenic and maintain the disease (Figure 1.4).

2 Dermatitis herpetiformis

Dermatitis herpetiformis (DH) is a distinct clinical entity associated with a gluten-sensitive enteropathy. Both the rash and the enteropathy are gluten-dependent and clear with gluten withdrawal.

EPIDEMIOLOGY

It is now generally accepted that all patients with dermatitis herpetiformis have associated gluten-sensitive enteropathy, although in many patients it is mild. Thus, areas with a high incidence of celiac disease (CD) also have a high incidence of DH, although CD appears to be five times more common than DH in the population where the disorders are prevalent.

CD is predominantly found in Caucasians, and the same applies to DH. The prevalence of DH has been reported to be 11.4 per 100 000 in Scotland[1] and Finland[2] and higher in Sweden, 19.6–39.2 per 100 000[3].

CD and DH outside Europe occur in the USA, Australia, New Zealand, Canada and Israel. However, these are all countries whose population is essentially Caucasian.

In one large series of DH patients[4] it was not found in Blacks, despite a large proportion of the population being Black. DH is extremely rare in Asians. In a 2-year review of subepidermal immunobullous disorders seen in Singapore, no patients with DH were found out of a total of 67[5]. DH has been reported in Japan[6] but the incidence was estimated to be 10–34 per 150 000 000, which is considerably less than that reported for European centers. There were also certain differences from DH found in Caucasians. First, the patients did not have the B8/DR3/DQ2 haplotype; of 12 patients who had intestinal biopsies, only three showed abnormalities; and in two patients who were tested for antiendomysial antibodies, none was detected. It is possible that 'DH' in the Japanese may be a variant of the DH seen in Caucasians, or may represent a different disorder.

ETIOLOGY

Genetics

It has been known for some time that CD tends to cluster in families, and that a genetic factor is likely to be involved. Because all patients with DH have CD it is therefore likely that DH has a genetic component involved in pathogenesis of the disease. Recent studies have looked at the genetics of both DH and CD to determine whether there is a common basis for the disorders, and what determines whether patients develop CD or DH.

Family studies

The most important family studies in DH have been carried out in Finland[7]. In a study of 1018 patients with DH, 999 were unrelated, and of these 105 (10.5%) had a first-degree relative with either DH (4.4%) or CD (6.1%). Thus, in first-degree relatives, there were approximately a similar number affected with CD and DH, implying a similar genetic background for both disorders.

In the propositi of DH patients the proportion who had an affected parent with either CD or DH was 13.6%, for siblings 18.7% and children 14.0%.

These figures suggest a Mendelian dominant mode of inheritance.

In another study from Finland[8], 380 patients with CD and 281 with DH had a total of 3158 first-degree relatives followed up for 14 years. It was found that 73 (19.2%) patients with CD and 51 (18.2%) with DH had affected first-degree relatives. The prevalence among relatives was similar for both diseases: 4.7% and 3.9% of the relatives had CD and 0.8% and 1.5% had DH, respectively. The annual incidence was 3 : 1000 relatives, which is 15 times that among the general population. CD and DH were mixed in several multiple-case families, implying a common genetic background.

Twin studies

Studies of monozygotic twins also suggest a common genetic basis for CD and DH. In a study of six monozygotic twins, three sets were concordant for DH, in two sets one had DH and one CD and in the sixth set one had CD and the other did not have CD or DH[9]. There have been two other reports of monozygotic twins in whom one had DH and the other CD[10,11]. These studies are conclusive evidence for a common genetic basis for CD and DH. Thus, it would appear that environmental factors may be important in determining whether patients develop DH or CD. It is known that in monozygotic twins the development of the immune system may be different due to the range of exposure to different antigens, which may be dietary or micro-organisms. Thus, whether individuals develop DH or CD may depend on immune responses which are different in DH subjects.

HLA studies

It has been known for nearly 30 years that there is a human leukocyte antigen (HLA) association with DH. The first reported association was with A1 and B8, and subsequently this was shown to be due to linkage with DR3, which in turn was due to linkage with DQ2. Two recent studies have shown that the DQ alleles A1*0501, B1*02, i.e. DQ2, and A1*03, B1*0302, i.e. DQ8, are present in patients with both DH and CD. In one study of DH patients the DQ2 allele was present in 43 of 50 (86%) and the DQ8 allele in six (12%) of the remaining seven patients[12]. In the other study, all 55 patients with DH and 201 of 212 (95%) CD patients had DQ2, and nine of the remaining 11 had DQ8[13]. These heterodimers of DQ2 and DQ8 have previously been shown to be present in CD and have now been shown to be present in DH in similar frequencies, which is further evidence of a common genetic basis for the two phenotypes of gluten sensitivity. However, it has recently been shown that, although there is evidence for a strong genetic component in CD, this is only partially accounted for by the HLA region[14]. This is evidence that CD and DH are polygenic disorders.

GENOME SCANS AND CANDIDATE GENES

To date there have been no published reports of genome scans in DH alone. However, results for DH have been included in a study of CD[15]. The first scan for CD was that in Irish families. Apart from the known HLA locus, the authors reported several possible candidate regions: 6p12, 3q27, 5q33.3, 7q31.3, 11p11, 15q26, 19p13.3, 19q13.4 and 22 cen. As with many polygenic disorders, confirmation from other studies does not always follow. There has been confirmation for 15q26[16] and 5q[17]. In a Finnish study, the patients were stratified into DH and CD. In the CD group, linkage to 2q33, but in the DH group to 5q and 11q, was reported. This is the first time that a genetic difference has been reported between CD and DH. Although previous studies have implied a common genetic basis, there may be additional modifying genes which may determine whether the individual develops DH or CD.

Microarray screen

A microarray screen for candidate genes in CD has recently been reported[18]. The two genes suggested by the author were prolyl endopeptidase (PREP) and TM4SF4. The PREP gene encodes a cytosolic prolyl endopeptidase that hydrolyzes proline-rich fragments such as gluten. PREP was found to be up-regulated in CD patients on a gluten-containing diet, compared with those on a gluten-free diet (GFD). The gene was up-regulated in controls taking gluten and was low in CD patients on a GFD. Thus, the presence of gluten in the intestine tends to up-regulate the PREP gene. It has been suggested that the enzyme function may be impaired in CD so that gluten is not broken down into small non-toxic peptides. Interestingly, it was proposed some 50 years ago that a failure of peptidases to digest gluten was the defect in CD.

Another candidate gene suggested by the microassay was TM4SF4. This gene plays an important part in the regulation of proliferation and differentiation of the epithelial cells. The study showed an eight-fold decrease in the level of TM4SF4 in CD duodenal biopsies compared with controls. One of the features of gluten-sensitive enteropathy is the increased mitosis and proliferation of the crypt epithelial cells and the subsequent lack of differentiation.

PATHOLOGY

It is not necessary to take a biopsy from a lesion to establish the diagnosis of DH. The presence of immunoglobulin A (IgA) in the uninvolved skin is the *sine qua non* for the diagnosis. The histological features are not specific for DH, and may be seen in other subepidermal blister diseases.

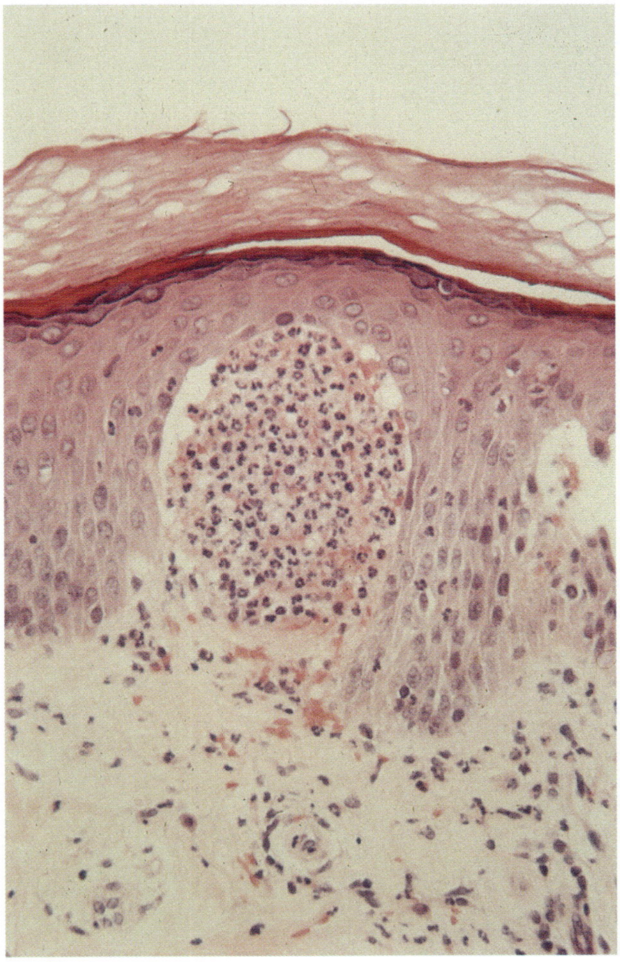

Figure 2.1 Dermal papillary microabscess in dermatitis herpetiformis

The histological features, however, are necessary for an understanding of the pathogenesis of DH and are described here. The initial lesion is a neutrophilic microabscess in the dermal papillae (Figure 2.1). These microabscesses coalesce to form a subepidermal blister (Figure 2.2). Neutrophils are the predominant cells in the blister, and leukocytoclasia and fibrin deposition are commonly seen. Eosinophils are present in 25% of blisters. In the dermis around the blood vessels there is a lymphohistiocytic cell infiltrate.

Skin biopsy: immunofluorescent studies

The presence of IgA in the upper dermis of uninvolved skin is the criterion for diagnosing DH. It is important to stress that the biopsy must be taken from uninvolved skin, as the immunoglobulins are destroyed in the actual skin lesions. It is customary to take the biopsy approximately 1 cm from an actual lesion. There are two patterns of IgA deposition in the skin. The first is so-called papillary (Figure 2.3) as the IgA is found in the dermal papillae and is usually seen as small 'dots' (granular) (Figure 2.4), but it may also be as linear streaks (fibrillar) (Figure 2.5). It is thought that those appearances are dependent on whether the connective tissue fibers are sectioned horizontally or vertically. The second pattern of IgA is along the line of the basement membrane and is termed 'linear' (Figures 2.6 and 2.7). However, there are breaks in the line and this pattern is termed linear granular, and must be distinguished from a homogeneous linear band of IgA along the line of the basement membrane as seen in linear IgA disease.

The papillary pattern of IgA deposition is the most common and is found in approximately 90% of

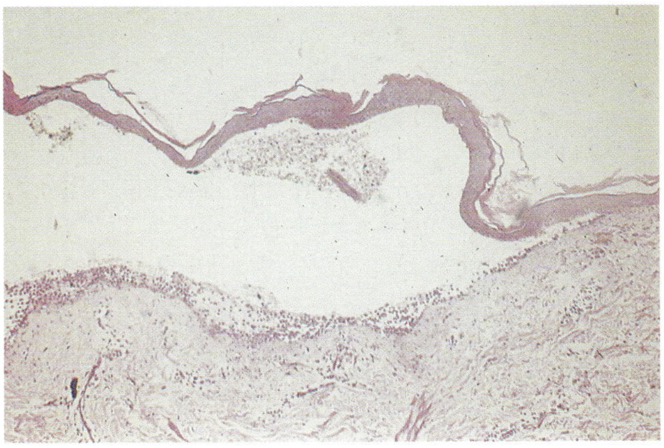

Figure 2.2 Subepidermal blister in dermatitis herpetiformis

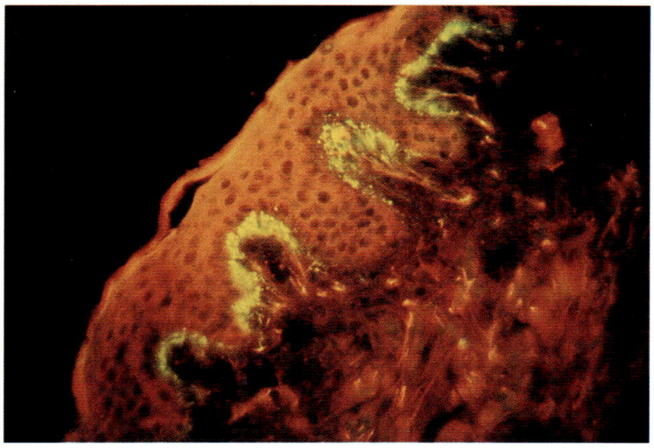

Figure 2.3 Immunoglobulin A (IgA) deposits in the dermal papillae in dermatitis herpetiformis (DH). The 'papillary pattern'

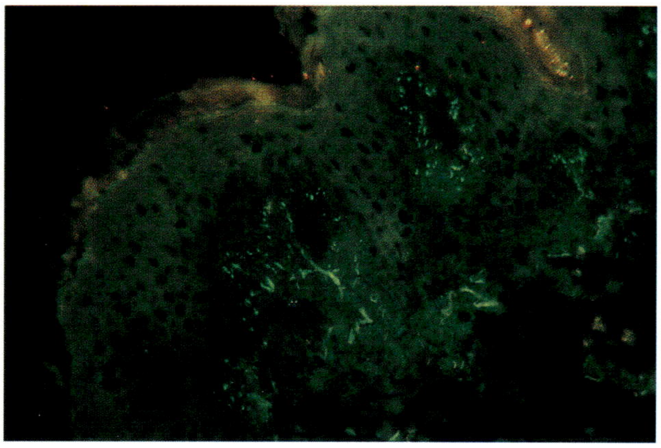

Figure 2.4 IgA deposits in DH appearing as 'granules': horizontal sectioning of 'fibers'

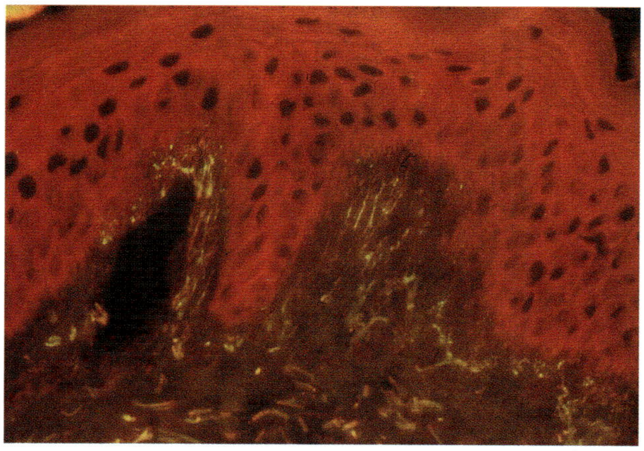

Figure 2.5 IgA deposits in dermal papillae with a 'fibrillar' appearance due to 'vertical' sectioning of 'fibers'

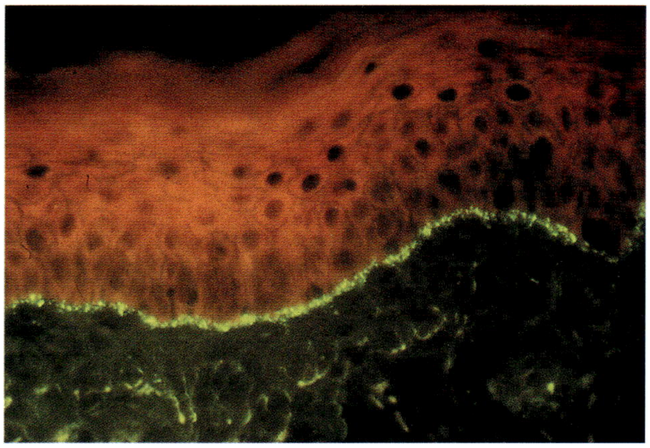

Figure 2.6 Linear granular deposition of IgA in DH. Although the pattern is essentially linear there are breaks and granules present

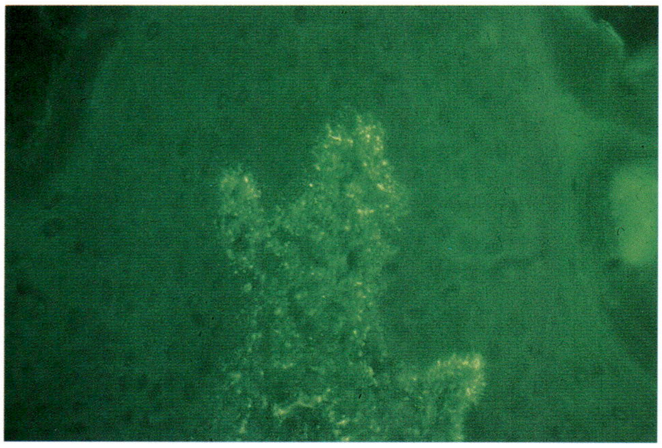

Figure 2.7 Combination of papillary IgA and linear IgA along the basement membrane region in DH

biopsies and the linear pattern in 10%. IgA is found in a single biopsy in approximately 95% of patients with DH. If no IgA is detected but the clinical suspicion for DH is high, then serial sections of the biopsy should be undertaken, and this will lead to detection in a further 3% of biopsies. If IgA is not found after serial sectioning then a second biopsy should be undertaken and this will prove positive in the remaining 2%. All patients with DH have IgA in the uninvolved skin, and the diagnosis of DH should not be made without its detection. In addition to IgA, complement C3, IgG and IgM may also be detected in the uninvolved skin, but the significance of this finding is unknown.

PATHOGENESIS

The original observations that patients with DH also had a gluten-sensitive enteropathy, and that the rash of DH cleared with a GFD, implicated gluten in the pathogenesis of DH[19]. However, what has not been explained is why one group of patients develops only an enteropathy (CD) and another group both an enteropathy and a skin eruption (DH). The demonstration that IgA deposits were present in the dermal papillae of uninvolved skin in DH and that patients with DH and CD had circulating IgA antibodies to reticulin[20] led to speculation about the pathogenesis of DH skin lesions. The localization of IgA to the site of reticulin in the dermis gave rise to the suggestion that binding of IgA to reticulin rendered it immunogenic and led to the development of antireticulin antibodies (ARAs). However, the incidence of ARAs was higher in patients with CD, and they did not have IgA in the skin. IgA antigliadin antibodies (AGAs) are also found in CD and DH, and it was suggested that an immune complex of IgA AGA/gliadin bound to reticulin in DH skin. Nevertheless, an explanation was lacking as to why these complexes bound to the reticulin of DH and not CD patients. The only suggestion was that the reticulin in DH patients was different from that found in CD, but this has never been substantiated. It was subsequently shown that gliadin binds to reticulin in the dermal papillae in both normal and DH skin (Figure 2.8)[21]. This was some support for a gliadin/antigliadin immune complex binding to the reticulin in DH skin. The incidence of ARAs was relatively low, being 20–25% in DH and 50% in CD. However,

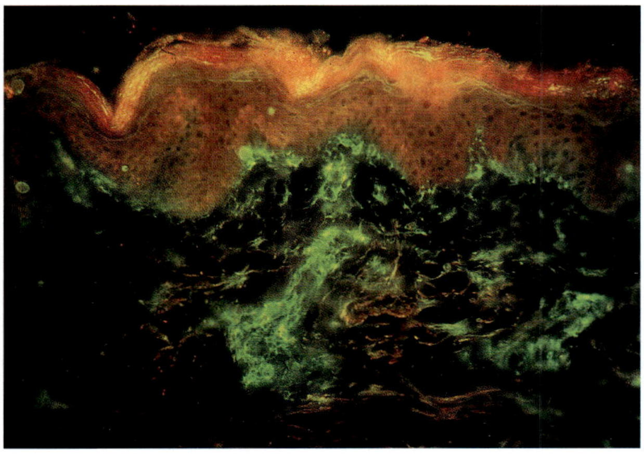

Figure 2.8 Gliadin binding to reticulin in the dermal papillae and upper dermis

using a different substrate (monkey esophagus) to detect circulating antibodies it was found that the incidence of a connective tissue antibody was 95% in CD and 70% in DH. The antibody was found to bind to connective tissue surrounding the muscle fibers, termed the endomysium, and the antibody was termed the antiendomysial antibody (AEMA).

The next major development was the demonstration that the autoantigen in CD was tissue-transglutaminase (tTG)[22], as it was possible to absorb out the AEMA with tTG. It was proposed that AEMA was a tissue-transglutaminase antibody (tTGA), and not one to a connective-tissue component. This concept was supported by the observation that there was a good correlation between the incidence of AEMA and tTGA in CD and DH. The incidence of tTGAs in CD is 93–97% and in DH 70–75%. The lower incidence in DH has been attributed to the milder enteropathy in DH.

tTG plays an important role in the cross-linking of connective-tissue fibers. This enzyme is found throughout the body and plays an active role in wound healing. tTG is synthesized by fibroblasts and keratinocytes and its primary role is stabilizing extracellular protein assemblies such as collagen fibrils, microfibrils, pericellular fibronectin matrix and basement membrane. In the healing skin, tTG is active in the dermal papillae and anchoring fibrils at the dermoepidermal junction. Interestingly, these are the sites of IgA deposition in DH. Type VII collagen is the major connective-tissue component of anchoring fibrils and is a potential substrate for tTG.

Although it has now been claimed that tTG is the autoantigen in CD, and antibodies to tTG are present in the circulation, how the enteropathy is produced has still to be elucidated. In addition, as patients with DH also have CD and tTGAs, do the latter play a role in the production of skin lesions?

As mentioned above, it has been shown that gliadin binds to reticulin in the skin. In addition, gliadin is a subtrate for tTG, so it is possible that gliadin is not binding to reticulin but to tTG, which is present predominantly at the sites of reticulin in the skin. It is also possible that gliadin is capable of binding to reticulin and tTG, and this will occur in the intestine as well as the skin. As a result of this binding, it has been suggested that neoepitopes are produced. These neoepitopes are presented to both T and B lymphocytes, by antigen-presenting cells, which in turn produce antibodies to tTG. In addition, these neoepitopes act as self-antigens and stimulate T cells to produce cytokines which damage the small intestine and produce the characteristic enteropathy seen in CD (Figure 2.9). One of the cytokines that is involved in the reversal of damage to cells and repair of connective tissue is transforming growth factor-β (TGF-β). However, tTG is necessary for the activation of TGF-β and this activation would be inhibited by tTGAs, and thus the connective tissue for maintenance of the villous architecture cannot be repaired (Figure 2.10). In addition, TGF-β is necessary for the activity of T suppressor cells, and is another factor in the continuing inflammation of the intestinal mucosa. However, there is no evidence that tTGAs interfere with the role of tTG at other sites of the body, i.e. repair of tissue in other organs following disease and trauma.

Another role for tTG in the enteropathy has been demonstrated. It has been shown that tTG deamidates gluten peptides. These deamidated peptides, compared with non-deamidated ones, produce a greater response by T-cell clones isolated from the intestine and reactive to gluten. It was shown that in the gluten peptides 134–153, the conversion of glutamine to glutamic acid at position 148 increased the binding of the peptide to HLA-DQ2, which then provoked a greater stimulatory response by gluten-sensitive T cells. This is in keeping with the requirement of a negatively charged anchor residue at position 148 for optimal bindings of the gliadin peptide to HLA-DQ2.

So what, if any, is the role of tTG in DH skin lesions? It is possible that a tTG/tTGA complex formed in the intestine could be carried to the skin where it is capable of binding to the sites of maximal tTG concentration in the skin, i.e. the dermal papillae and anchoring fibrils of the basement membrane. If T cells primed to react to neoepitopes of tTG (produced in the intestine) arrived in the skin,

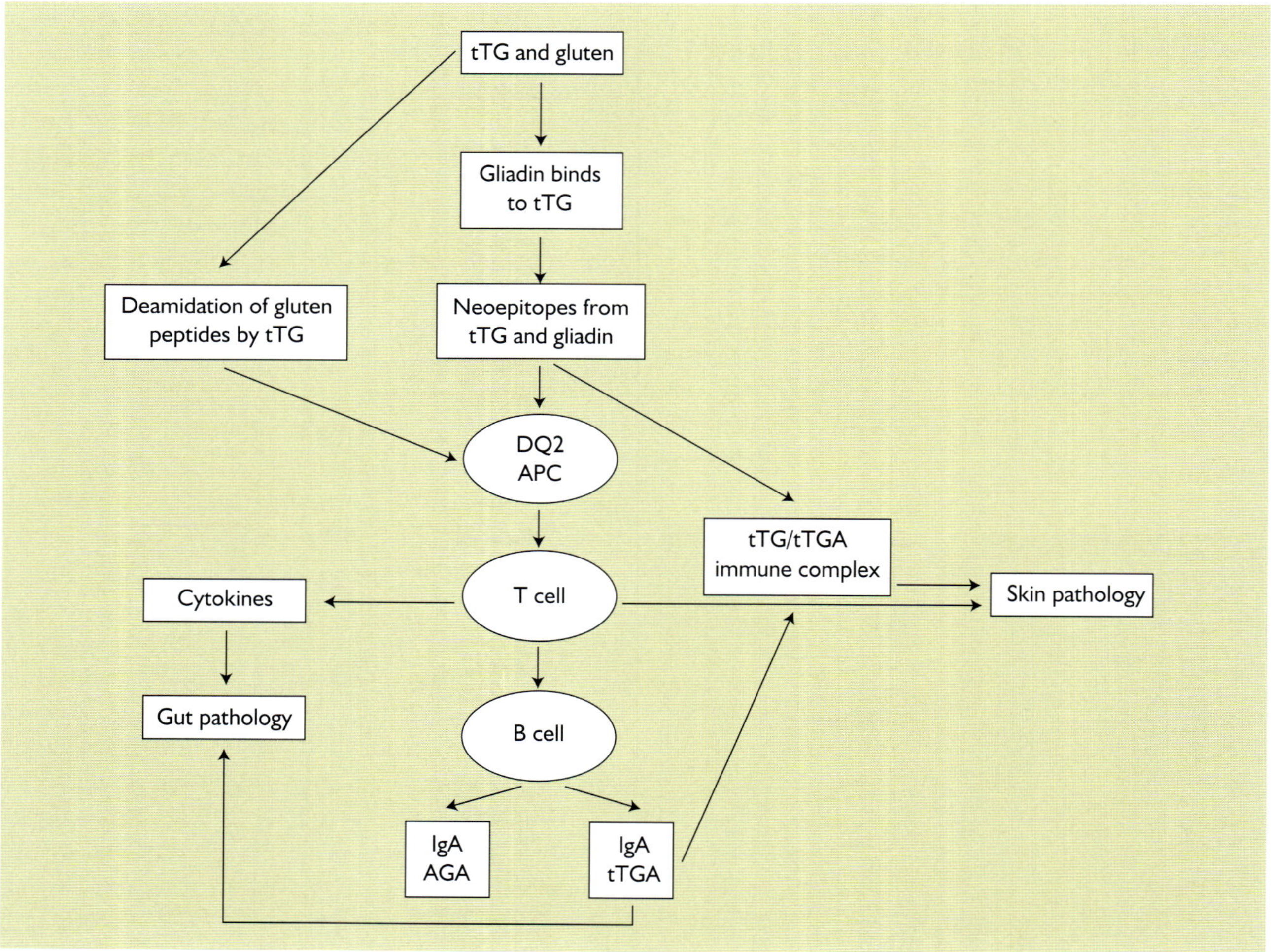

Figure 2.9 Possible pathways for skin and gut pathology in DH. tTG, tissue-transglutaminase; tTGA, tissue-transglutaminase antibodies; AGA, antigliadin antibodies; APC, antigen-presenting cell; IgA, immunoglobulin A

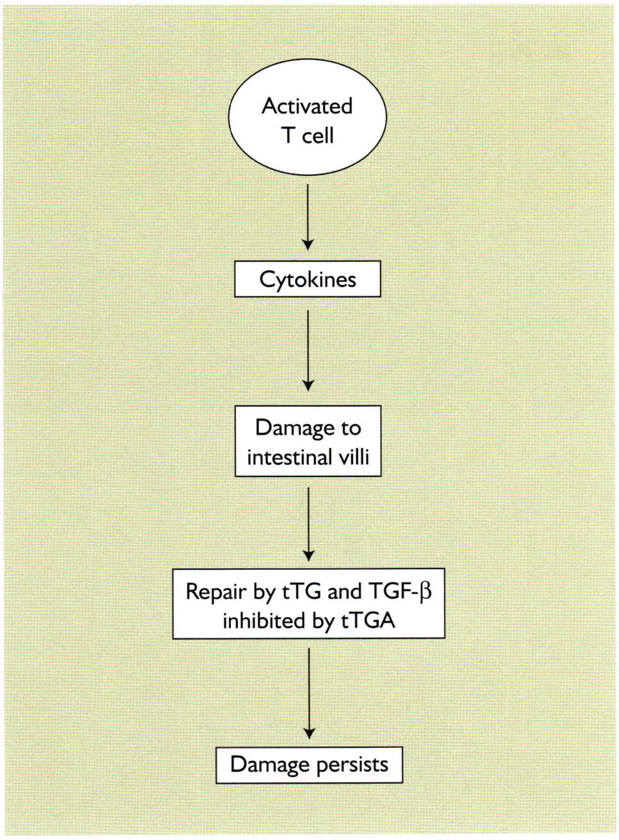

Figure 2.10 Pathogenesis of intestinal lesion. tTG, tissue-transglutaminase; TGF-β, transforming growth factor-β; tTGA, tissue-transglutaminase antibodies

they could be activated by the tTG/tTGA complex. Alternatively, it is possible that tTGAs produced in the gut could bind to the tTG in the skin, which in turn damages the tTG which results in the formation of neoepitopes to be recognized by T cells primed for these peptides in the gut (Figure 2.11).

Recently it has been claimed[23] that transglutaminase type 3 or epidermal transglutaminase (TG3) is the autoantigen in DH. In the skin, TG3 is found in the epidermis, the highest concentration being in the upper epidermis, and its function is to help in production of the cornified envelope assembly, i.e. formation of the stratum corneum. TG3 is not present in the dermis[24]. It has been shown that in addition to IgA tTGAs, antibodies to IgA TG3 are present both in DH and CD sera[23]. However, in DH there is a higher avidity of the antibody directed against TG3. In addition, although antibodies to TG3 are present in the sera of both CD and DH patients, the concentration of TG3A was found to be higher in DH than in CD. The same authors also showed that TG3 was present in the IgA aggregates in the skin, and speculated that there was cross-reactivity between tTGAs and TG3As. The authors' hypothesis was that after prolonged gliadin provocation, specific cross-reacting antibodies develop in patients who will progress to DH. These antibodies have a low affinity for tTG but

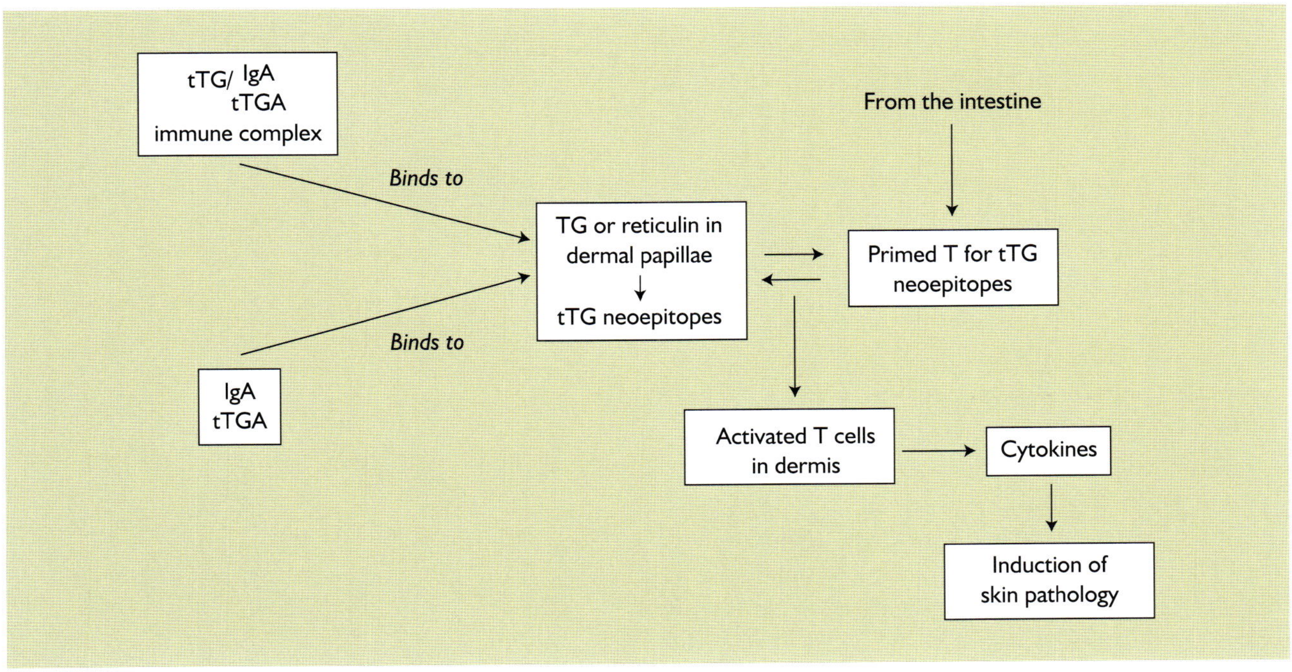

Figure 2.11 Scheme for IgA deposition and activated T cells in the skin. See Figures 2.9 and 2.10 for definitions

an extremely high affinity for TG3. Whether they arise against TG3 as a primary antigen or are the result of epitope spreading is unknown.

There are several unanswered questions in this hypothesis. First, why is it that only DH patients develop these cross-reacting antibodies? Prolonged gliadin provocation cannot be the reason, as there are many CD patients with mild or 'latent' disease who also have prolonged gliadin provocation without progressing to DH. TG3 is found in the epidermis and not the dermis. The reason for developing antibodies to TG3 has not been explained. It is possible that it is secondary to the skin lesions in DH that cause damage to the epidermis with release of TG3 or TG3 neoepitopes which result in the development of antibodies. The observation that TG3As are lower in CD than in DH may be due to the fact that CD patients do not have skin lesions.

One might also argue that TG3As do not appear to be pathogenic. If they were, then there should be damage to the stratum corneum, as TG3 is necessary to maintain the cornified envelope.

The role of the IgA aggregates (whether they contain TG3 or not) in the skin of DH patients has not been satisfactorily explained. It should be stressed that the IgA is found in all the uninvolved skin and that it is still present in the skin for many years after control of the rash with a gluten-free diet (GFD). It is also present in the skin of DH patients in spontaneous remission. It has even been suggested that the IgA in the skin in DH is an epiphenomenon, and not important in the pathogenesis of the skin lesions. At present it is appropriate to say that the role, if any, of IgA in the skin in DH patients has yet to be elucidated.

In discussion of the pathogenesis of DH it should be remembered that the presence of IgA in the skin is only one factor. The production of the skin lesion is dependent on several other factors. A lymphocytic/histiocytic infiltrate in the dermis is an early feature. A perivascular infiltrate of T lymphocytes, both CD4 and CD8, is present (Figure 2.12). This infiltrate is seen in uninvolved skin but to a greater extent in involved lesional skin. The T cells, however, are not gluten-specific.

There is increased expression of interleukin-8 (IL-8) (Figure 2.13) in the basal keratinocytes of lesional DH skin, and of granulocyte-macrophage colony-stimulating factor (GM-CSF) (Figure 2.14) in the dermoepidermal dendritic cells. There is also an increase of endothelial cell–leukocyte adhesion

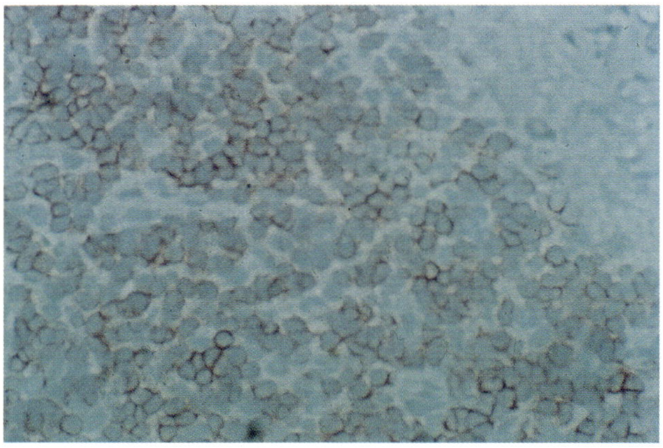

Figure 2.12 CD3 T-cell infiltrate in the dermis of lesional DH skin

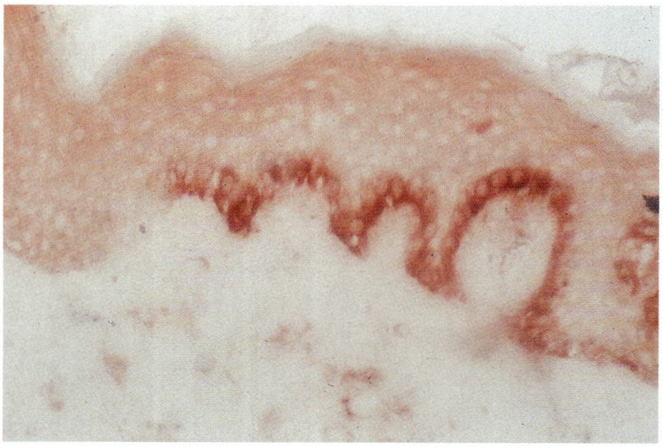

Figure 2.13 Interleukin-8 (IL-8) in the basal keratinocytes in lesional DH skin

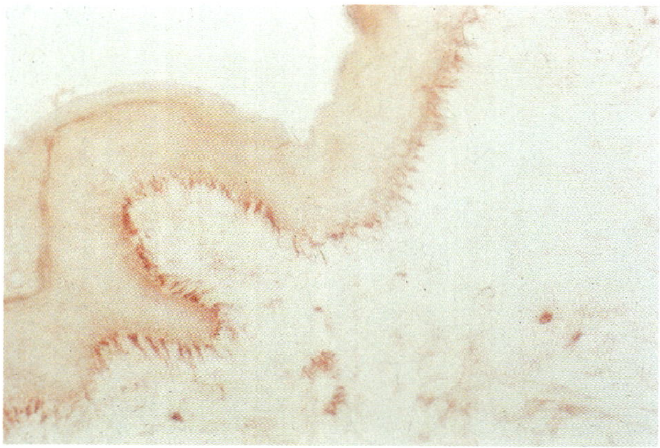

Figure 2.14 Granulocyte–macrophage colony-stimulating factor (GM-CSF) expressed by dendritic cells at the dermoepidermal junction in DH

molecule-1 (ELAM-1) expression in the deep dermal network and subpapillary dermis of lesional DH skin. These cytokine findings are compatible with the influx of neutrophils into the skin in DH, as IL-8 is a strong chemoattractant for neutrophils. GM-CSF stimulates the expression of IgA Fc receptors on neutrophils and will allow binding of the neutrophils to the IgA. This in turn leads to activation of the neutrophils with the release of enzymes responsible for blister formation (Figure 2.15). These observations and sequence of events explain the development of a DH skin lesion with IgA involved, but it is not the initiating factor. However, what induces the increased expression of ELAM-1, IL-8 and GM-CSF has not been elucidated. It has been suggested that it may be trauma to the skin, as DH lesions tend to occur at pressure points, e.g. elbows and buttocks.

Although several observations have been made regarding the possible pathogenesis of DH, it is reasonable to conclude that at present the answer as to how gluten causes the skin lesions is speculative. In addition, a valid explanation of why some patients with gluten sensitivity develop skin lesions (DH) and why some do not (CD) is still awaited.

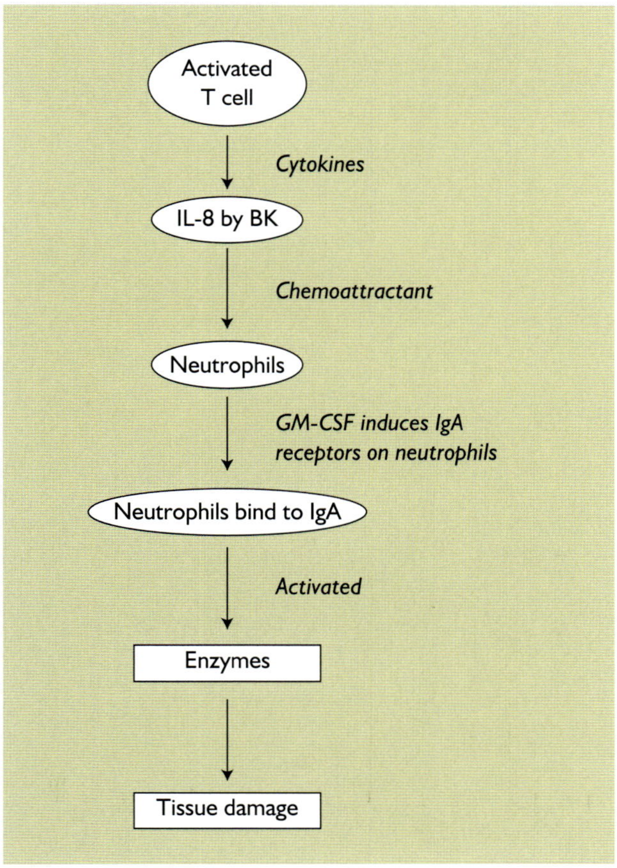

Figure 2.15 Pathogenesis of blister formation in the skin in DH. BK, basal keratinocyte; IL-8, interleukin-8; GM-CSF, granulocyte–macrophage colony-stimulating factor

CLINICAL FEATURES

Sex incidence

Overall, DH is slightly more common in males (3 : 2). However, under the age of 20 years it is more common in females (3 : 2).

Age of onset

DH most commonly presents in late adolescence and early adult life (15–40 years). However, it may present in infancy and childhood, the youngest recorded being 10 months[25], or at any age in adult life, the oldest recorded being over 90 years[3].

Morphology

The typical lesions of DH are red urticarial papules, plaques, blisters (Figures 2.16–2.21) and excoriations (Figures 2.22 and 2.23). The blisters vary in size from 2–3 mm to 1–2 cm. They usually arise from the urticarial plaques, but can also arise from normal-looking skin. The lesions are often grouped (Figures 2.19 and 2.24), and hence the term herpetiformis. DH is one of the most irritating skin disorders, and thus patients excoriate the lesions. This results in the blisters being broken at an early stage, and they may not be present when the patient is seen (Figures 2.22, 2.23 and 2.27). It is in fact more common to see scabs and crusted papules at the site of previous blister formation than to see actual blisters. Thus, the distribution of the rash (see below) may be more important than the appearance of the eruption in suggesting the diagnosis.

Distribution

The eruption of DH tends to be symmetrical (Figures 2.19, 2.20, 2.24, 2.25 and 2.27). The commonest site for the eruption is the extensor surface of the elbows and proximal third of the forearm (Figures 2.19–2.23). This site is affected in over 90% of patients. The second commonest site is the buttock, and is involved in presentation in 70% of patients (Figures 2.24–2.26). Although the extensor surface of the knees (Figures 2.27 and 2.28) is listed as the third commonest site, it is involved only in approxi-

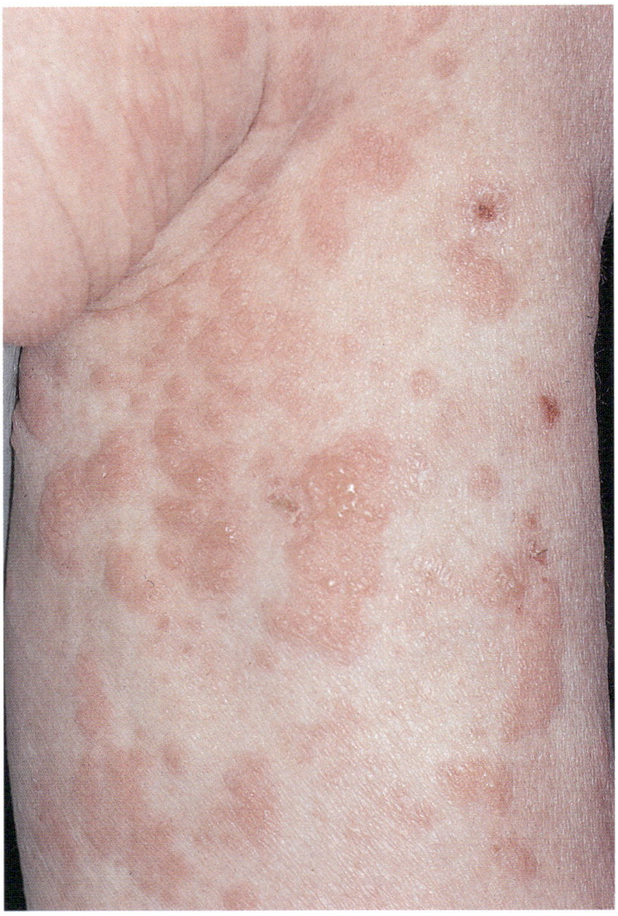

Figure 2.16 Urticarial plaques on the trunk and upper arm with a small blister. Early stage of DH

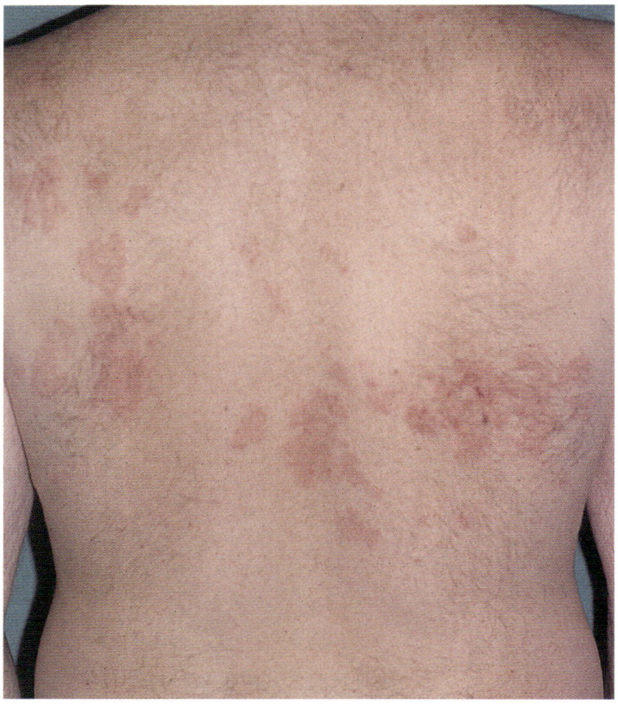

Figure 2.17 Urticarial patches on the back in DH

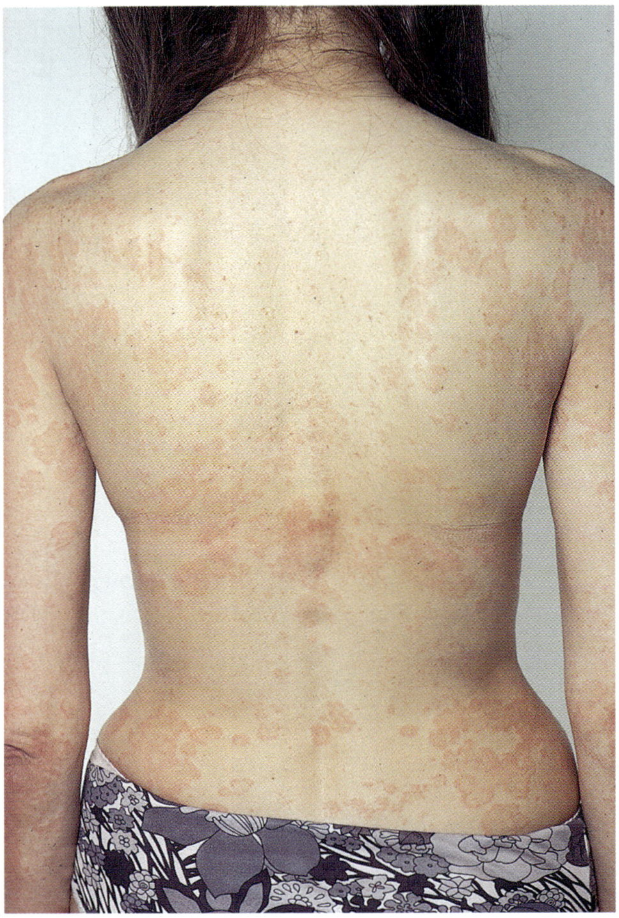

Figure 2.18 Extensive urticarial lesions on the back and arms in active DH

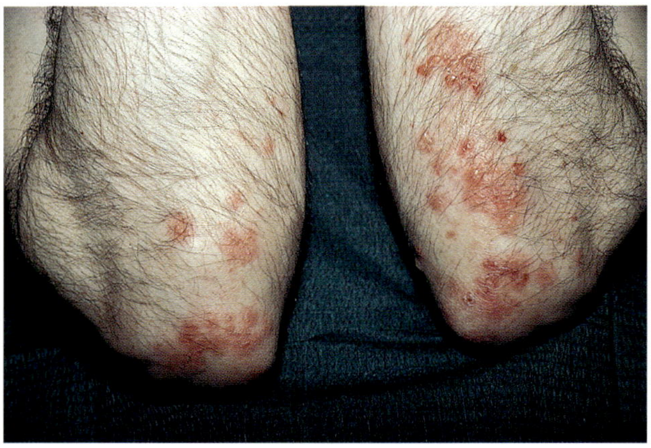

Figure 2.19 Blisters and urticarial plaques on the elbows and proximal forearms in DH

mately one-third of patients. Although the extensor surfaces of the knees and elbows are the common sites for involvement, lesions may also be seen in the flexures of these joints (Figures 2.29 and 2.30).

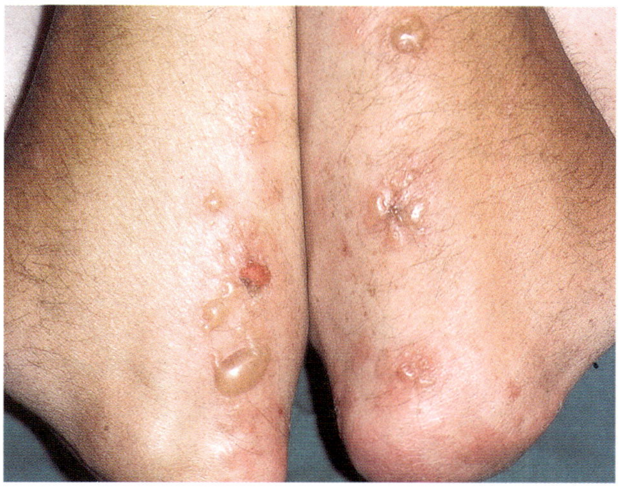

Figure 2.20 Grouped lesions in DH: small blisters on an urticarial base

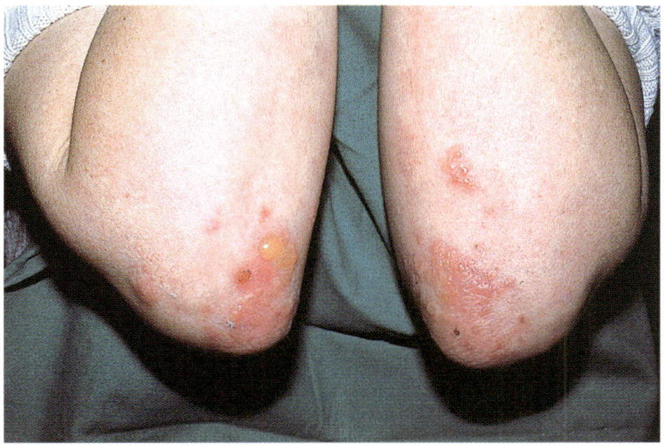

Figure 2.21 Symmetrical urticarial plaques and blisters on the elbows in DH

Involvement at these sites is often diagnosed as atopic eczema.

The eruption of DH may occur anywhere except for the palms and soles. The face, neck and scalp (Figures 2.31 and 2.32) are often involved, but later in the course of the disorder rather than at the beginning. In addition, when there is a flare-up of the eruption, for whatever reason, the face and scalp are frequently affected. Occasionally the eruption is widespread, with involvement of the trunk (Figures 2.33–2.35), limbs and face. This may lead to difficulty in diagnosis for the inexperienced physician.

The lesions may also present at sites of pressure, e.g. from clothing, bra straps (Figure 2.36) and tight belts.

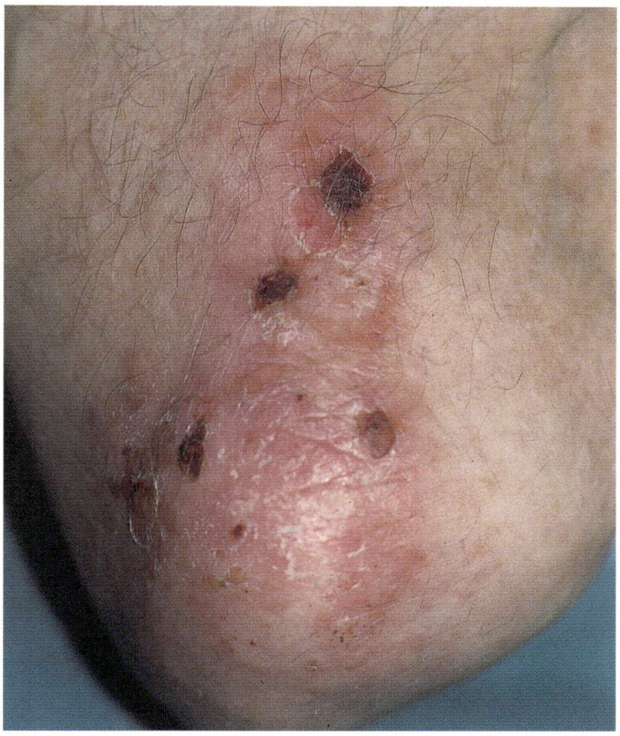

Figure 2.22 Excoriations at sites of previous blisters on the elbow

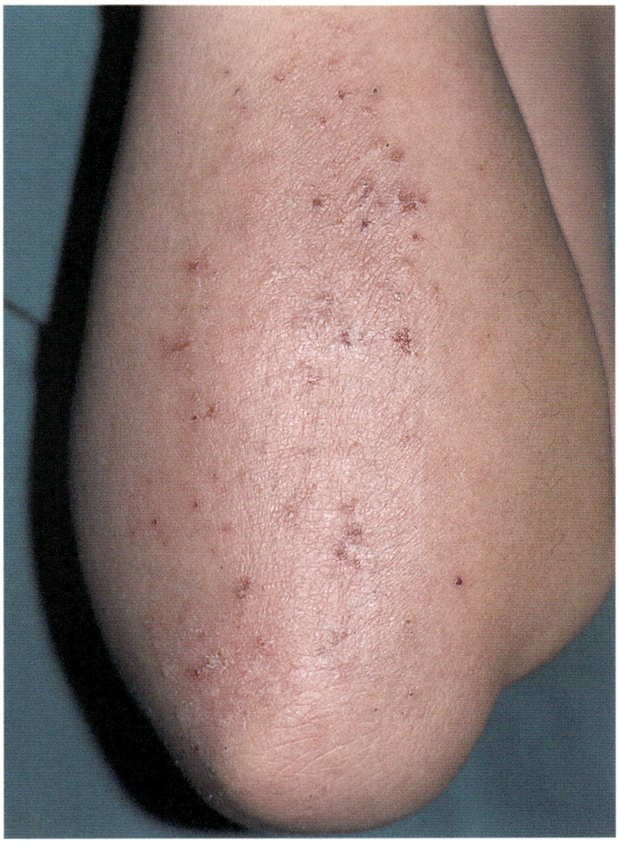

Figure 2.23 Excoriated extensor forearm: no blisters present

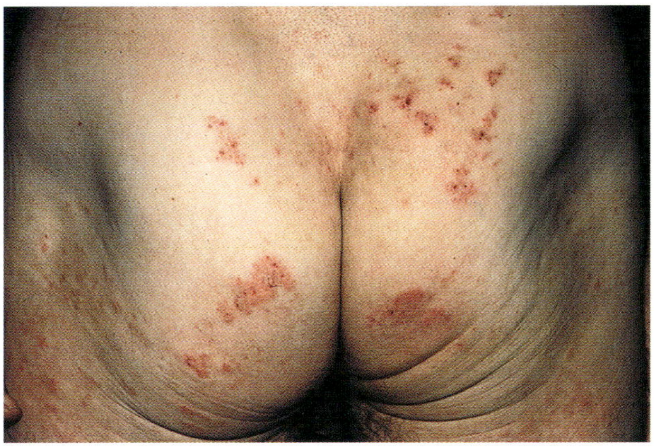

Figure 2.24 Grouped symmetrical lesions on buttocks

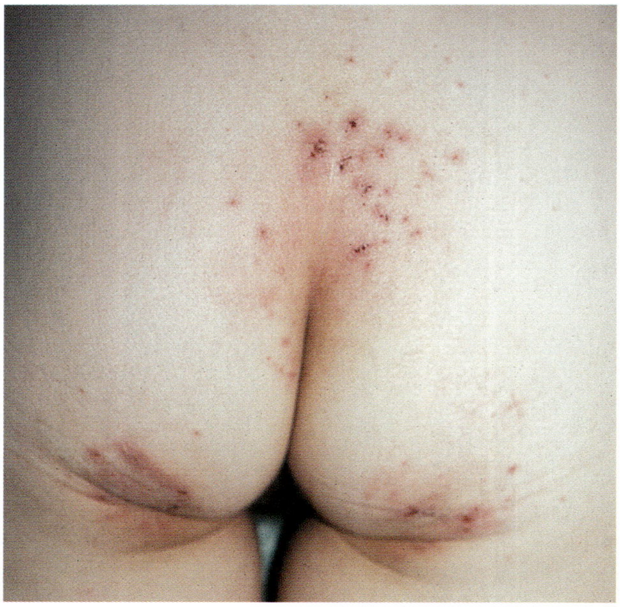

Figure 2.25 Symmetrical lesions on buttocks in DH

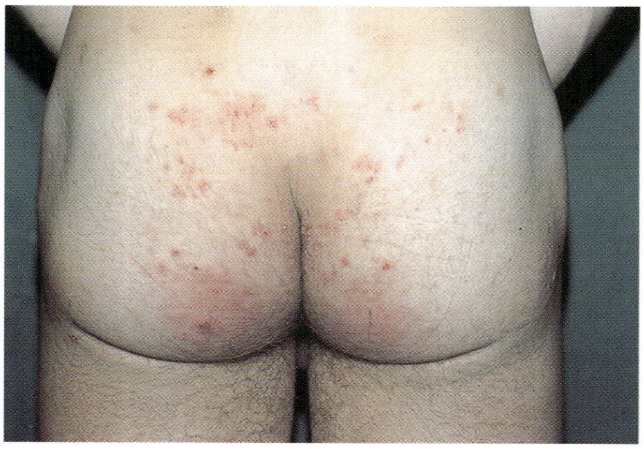

Figure 2.26 Symmetrical group of papules on the buttocks. Blisters are rarely seen at this site

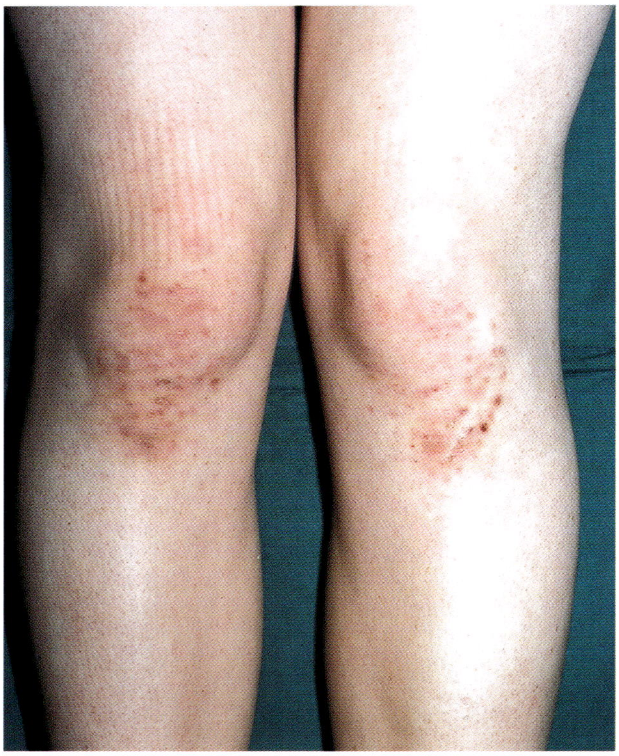

Figure 2.27 Excoriated papules on the knees in DH

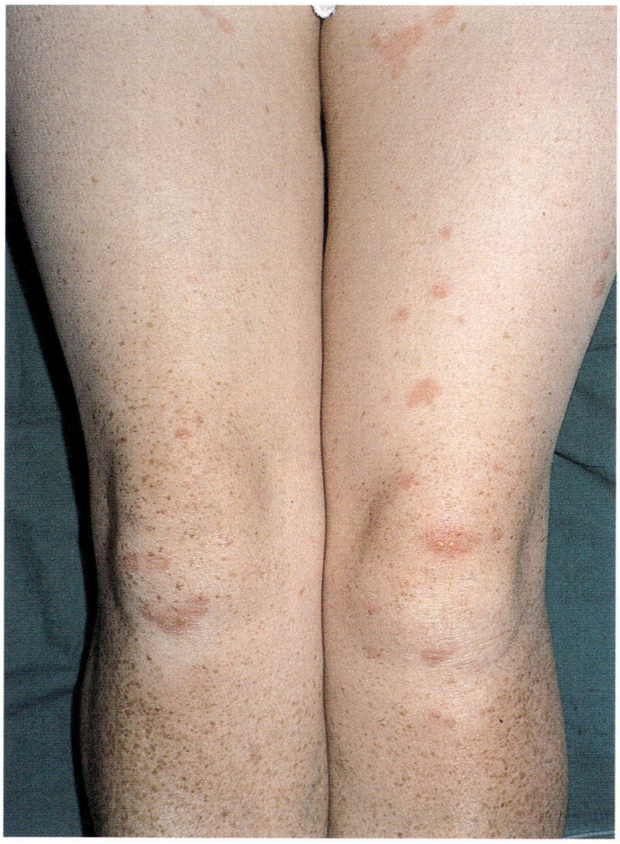

Figure 2.28 Urticarial plaques, extensor surface of knees and thighs

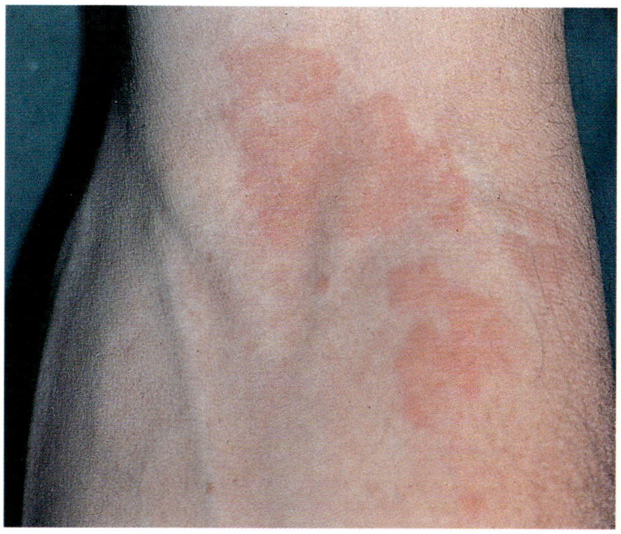

Figure 2.29 Urticarial plaques on the antecubital fossae in DH: often confused with atopic eczema but there is no scaling in DH

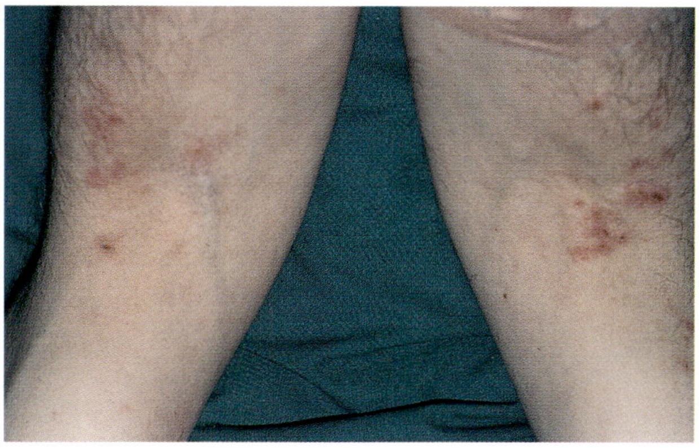

Figure 2.30 Grouped excoriated papules on the antecubital fossae in DH

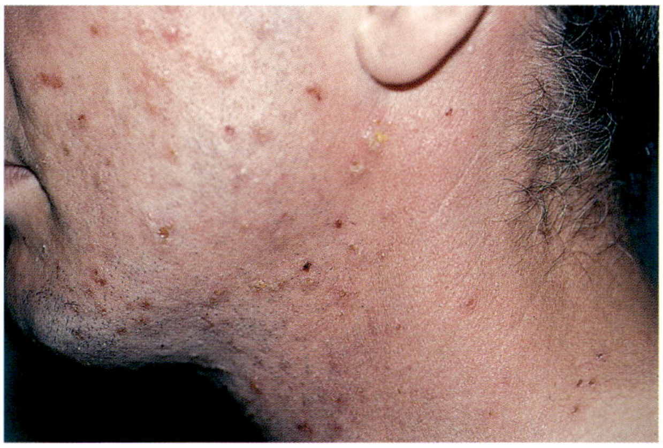

Figure 2.31 Excoriated papules on the face and neck. Two pustules are present due to secondary infection. This presentation is often misdiagnosed as excoriated eczema or folliculitis

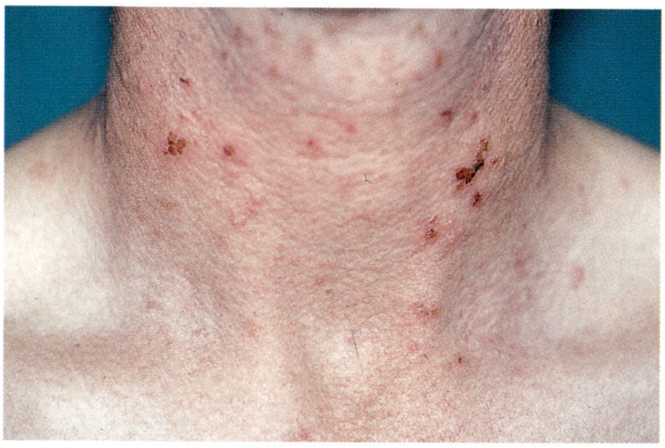

Figure 2.32 Excoriations and red papules on the neck. The common sites for the eruption should be examined otherwise the diagnosis of DH will be missed

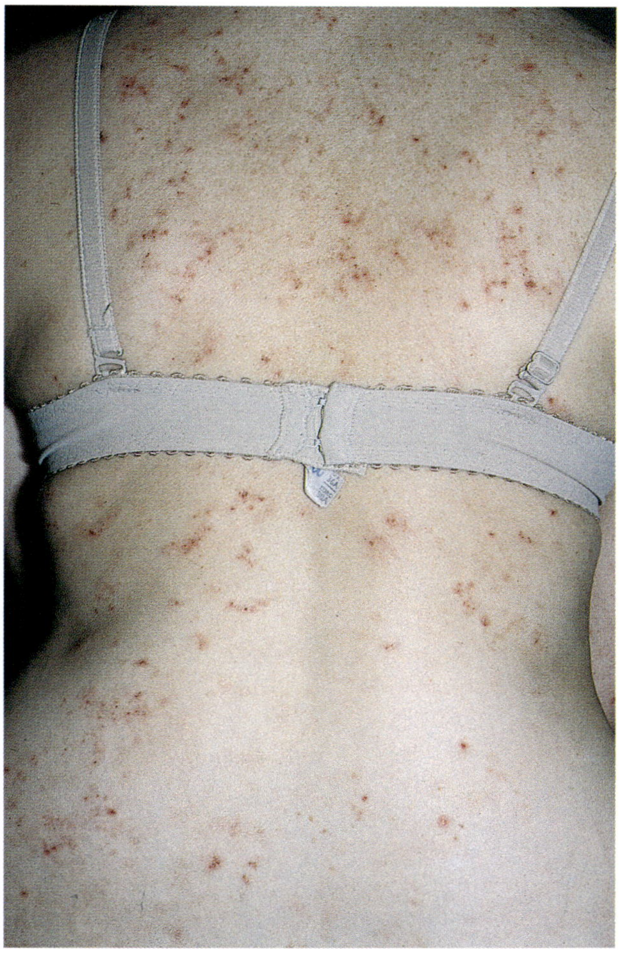

Figure 2.33 Extensive eruption on the back in DH. Some of the lesions appear to be grouped

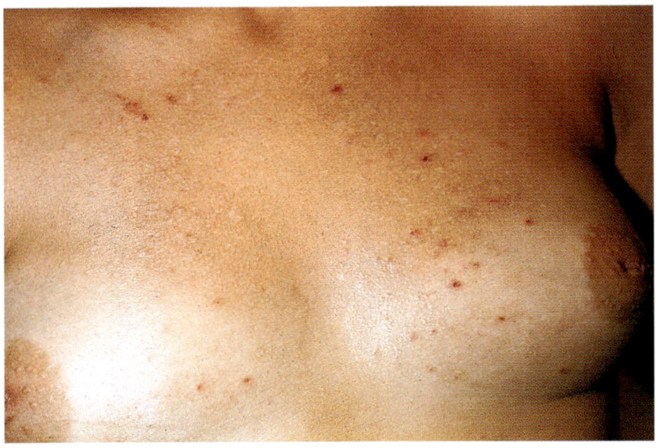

Figure 2.34 Scattered excoriated papules on the chest in DH. It is difficult to make the diagnosis without more classical lesions

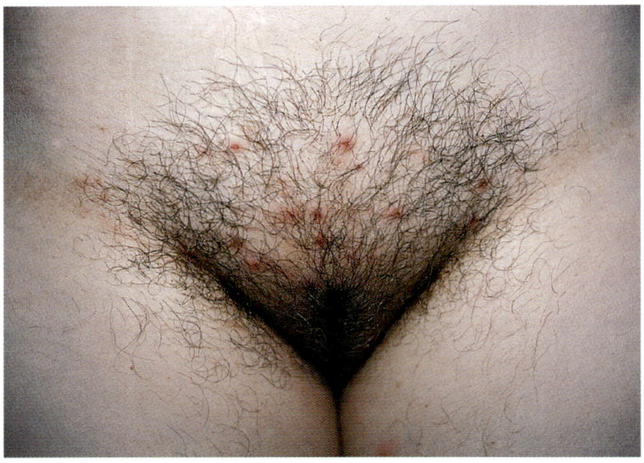

Figure 2.35 Papular eruption in pubic area in DH: will be confused with scabies, pediculosis pubis

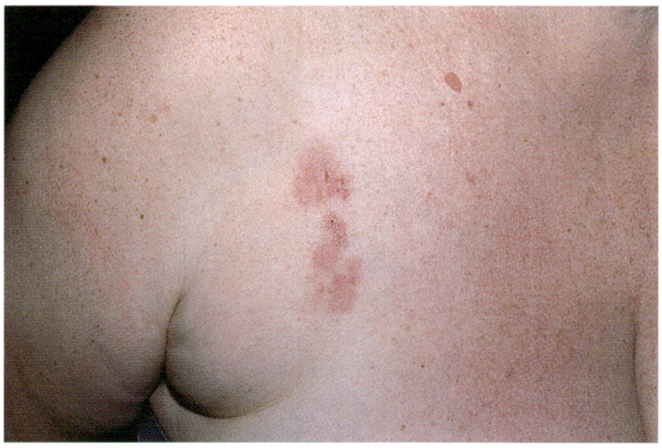

Figure 2.36 Grouped red plaques at site of pressure from bra strap

INVESTIGATIONS

As DH is associated with gluten-sensitive enteropathy (GSE) and autoimmune disorders, several investigations are necessary once the diagnosis has been made and on follow-up.

Hematological

A full blood count is mandatory. Anemia may be present due to iron and folate malabsorption, and during treatment with dapsone because of hemolysis. Macrocytosis may be present due to folate deficiency or B12 deficiency, the latter associated with pernicious anemia, or due to hemolysis related to dapsone treatment. The appropriate tests for folate, B12 and iron status should be carried out if indicated. The peripheral blood-film may show the presence of Howell–Jolly bodies indicating splenic atrophy, which is found in DH and celiac disease.

Biochemistry

Liver function tests have been found to be abnormal in 17% of patients with DH[26]. However, the most common cause of a raised bilirubin level is hemolysis from dapsone treatment and not liver disease *per se*. Abnormal liver function tests may be due to associated autoimmune liver disease. In addition, abnormal liver function tests are associated non-specifically with GSE and they revert to normal with gluten withdrawal from the diet. Blood glucose may be raised due to associated type I diabetes. Rarely, a low calcium level may be found if there is severe malabsorption.

Autoantibody screening

As mentioned above, there is a significant increase in autoimmune disorders in association with DH. The commonest disorders are thyroid disease, pernicious anemia and type I diabetes. Thyroid and gastric parietal cell antibodies should be looked for routinely. Although the incidence of autoimmune connective-tissue diseases is considerably lower, there is an increase, and screening for antinuclear antibodies should be carried out. Other autoantibodies should only be looked for if there is a specific clinical indication, e.g. antimitochondrial, antiacetylcholine receptor.

Antireticulin (ARAs), antiendomysial (AEMAs) and tissue-transglutaminase antibodies (tTGAs) are not necessary for the diagnosis of DH; this depends on the presence of IgA deposits in the skin. However, their presence is supportive evidence for the diagnosis, and may also be helpful in unraveling the pathogenesis of DH. The incidence of ARAs is relatively low in DH (20%), but is considerably higher for AEMAs (75%) and tTGAs (70–75%). These figures are lower than those found for CD, and probably reflect the severity of the enteropathy in the two diseases.

Small-intestinal biopsy

Although the criterion for diagnosing DH is the presence of IgA in the uninvolved skin, a small-intestinal biopsy should be performed. If patients are to be treated with a GFD then a baseline biopsy is helpful. The small-intestinal biopsy is still the 'gold standard' for diagnosing and staging gluten-sensitive enteropathy. Although both AEMAs and tTGAs have a high specificity for gluten-sensitive enteropathy, the incidence in DH is only 70–75%. Villous atrophy (equivalent to flat or convoluted macroscopic appearance) (Figure 2.37) is seen in only two-thirds of DH patients on a single biopsy. However, other features indicative of gluten-sensitive enteropathy are present. In addition, it has been shown that if multiple biopsies are taken from the upper small intestine, the incidence of villous atrophy rises to 95%. Even if villous atrophy is not present in DH patients, intestinal biopsy shows an increase of intraepithelial lymphocytes. The average number of intraepithelial lymphocytes in the normal small intestine is approximately 150 per 1000 epithelial cells, whilst in CD and DH patients it is 450. This increase in intraepithelial lymphocytes is the same irrespective of the macroscopic appearance of the small intestine, i.e. whether there is a flat mucosal surface or one exhibiting normal villi with finger-like processes (Figure 2.38). In addition, there is an increase in gamma–delta ($\gamma\delta$) T lymphocytes in the intestinal mucosa in gluten-sensitive enteropathy, and which is seen in DH patients. Although the morphological features and intraepithelial lymphocyte count return to normal with a GFD, the increase in gamma–delta T lymphocytes is not affected by gluten withdrawal. Approximately 5% of patients have intestinal biopsies showing normal morphology and no increase in the intraepithelial lymphocytes. However, gluten challenge will result in the induction of villous atrophy and an increase in the intraepithelial lymphocytes. Thus, in all DH patients it is possible to demonstrate features of GSE, although in some they are mild.

NATURAL HISTORY AND PROGNOSIS

DH in the majority of individuals tends to be a persistent disorder. In patients not treated with a GFD and followed up for 25 years the spontaneous remission rate was 10–15%[27,28]. In patients whose eruption was completely controlled with a GFD for longer than 10 years, the eruption returned on reintroduction of gluten in 11 of 12 (92%) patients. This implies that the basic pathogenetic mechanisms are not altered by a GFD. The spontaneous remission rate is similar when the eruption is controlled by drugs or gluten exclusion. In some patients the eruption tends to be less severe as the individuals

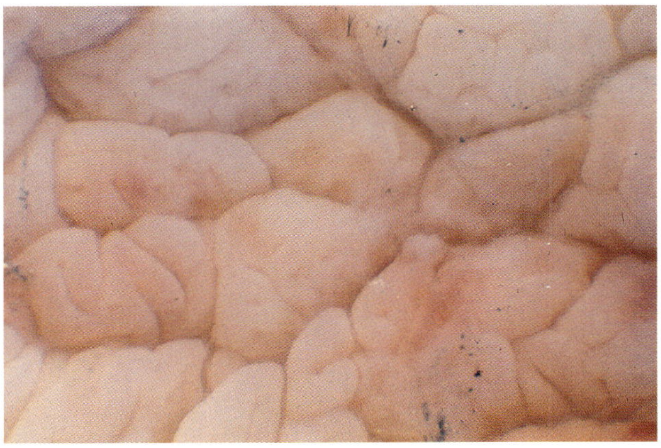

Figure 2.37 A flat intestinal mucosa equivalent to villous atrophy on histological sections

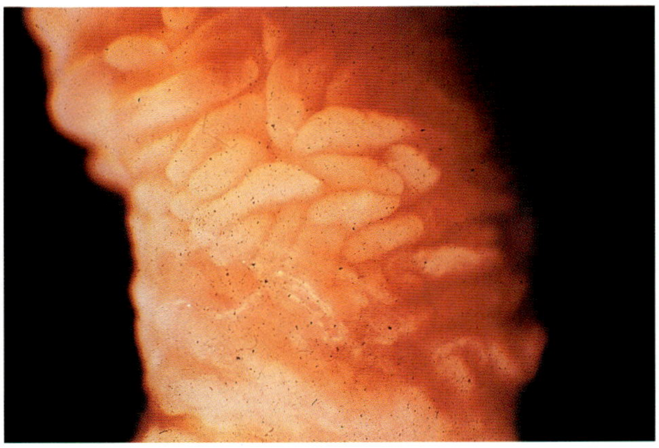

Figure 2.38 A normal intestinal mucosa. The villi appear as fingers and leaf-like projections

become older. There is also a suggestion that the rash is less severe in those individuals with late onset of the skin lesions[3].

MANAGEMENT

The eruption of DH can be controlled by drugs and by a GFD. Drugs can bring relief from the irritation quickly (a few days), whilst a GFD takes on average 6 months before any benefit occurs. Thus, a GFD should be introduced once the diagnosis has been established and appropriate drug therapy commenced at the same time. The drugs which are used in DH are dapsone, sulfapyridine and sulfamethoxypyridazine. These drugs have a very rapid action in DH, and may relieve irritation within 48 hours and clear the rash after 1 week. However, the converse also occurs, with the irritation returning within 24 hours and the rash within 2–3 days of discontinuing the drugs. The mechanism of action of the current drugs in DH is thought to involve the migration, activation and binding of neutrophils to the IgA in the skin.

Dapsone

Dapsone was first introduced for the treatment of DH in 1950. The initial dose of dapsone is 100 mg daily, and the patient should reattend 2 weeks later. If the rash is completely controlled then the dose should be reduced to 50 mg daily. Further reduction in dosage should be attempted if the rash remains clear by increasing the interval of time between each dose, i.e. first to alternate days, then every third day and by further increments of a day until a schedule of once a week is reached. At this dosage it is unlikely that the patient requires dapsone. If control of the rash is not achieved, the dose may be increased to 200 mg daily and then by 100 mg daily every 2 weeks until a dose of 400 mg daily is reached. If no control is achieved, then the diagnosis of DH should be reviewed, including a second biopsy for detecting IgA in the uninvolved skin.

Hemolysis is one of the commonest side-effects and will occur to some extent in most patients. The degree of hemolysis varies between patients; in some it may be severe, with a sharp fall in hemoglobin concentration, and this will necessitate discontinuing dapsone. Hemolysis occurs early after starting the drug, and thus it is important to see the patient within 2 weeks and repeat the full blood count and also do a reticulocyte count. If severe hemolysis does not occur at the beginning of treatment, the length of time between follow-up appointments can be gradually lengthened, and at each visit the hematological parameters should be ascertained. Even patients established on dapsone should be seen at least every 6 months. If patients, or their ancestors, come from the Middle East it is important to establish that these patients are not glucose-6-phosphate dehydrogenase deficient. If they are, then dapsone should not be used. Deficiency of this enzyme will lead to severe hemolysis.

Methemoglobinemia is another common side-effect of dapsone, and presents as cyanosis. The degree of cyanosis is not directly related to the dose of dapsone. The importance of methemoglobinemia is that it will reduce the oxygen-carrying capacity of the blood. Unless severe, methemoglobinemia is not a problem in the young and middle-aged, but in the elderly there may be impaired cardiac and/or cerebral blood flow, which does not cause symptoms but may if the oxygen-carrying capacity of the blood is reduced.

Headache, lethargy, insomnia and depression are not uncommon side-effects, and if severe the dapsone should be discontinued. Agranulocytosis is a rare but a recognized side-effect.

Peripheral neuropathy, which is usually a mononeuritis of the entrapment type, is a rare but well-recognized side-effect.

Approximately 25% of patients taking dapsone will experience side-effects which warrant discontinuing the drug. Other drugs are available and should be substituted.

Sulfapyridine

The initial dose is 2.0 g daily. The patient should be seen after 2 weeks and the dose adjusted according to the clinical response. The maximum dose is 4.0 g daily and the lowest dose may be as low as 0.5 g daily.

Side-effects are nausea, lethargy and depression. Rarely, agranulocytosis, hemolytic anemia, renal calculi and central nervous system abnormalities may occur.

Sulfamethoxypyridazine

This is a relatively unknown sulfonamide, but a valuable option for the treatment of DH. The initial dose is 1.0 g per day and the dosage range is 0.5–1.5 g daily.

Side-effects, which are uncommon, include drug rash, nausea, lethargy and agranulocytosis.

Choice of drug

The choice of drug for treating DH and other bullous disorders is often a personal one. Dapsone is relatively cheap and readily available, but has a high incidence of side-effects. Sulfapyridine and sulfamethoxypyridazine are now 'orphan drugs', and more difficult to obtain and relatively expensive. However, the incidence of side-effects is relatively less than with dapsone. A disadvantage of sulfapyridine is the large number of tablets to be taken each day. (The tablets are 0.5 g, and some patients require 4.0 g daily.)

Combination therapy

If an increase of dosage of a particular drug to obtain control of the rash is precluded by side-effects, it is possible to combine any of the three drugs to obtain an increased therapeutic effect.

Other drugs

Very occasionally, patients cannot take dapsone or sulfonamides, and will require drug therapy before the benefit of a GFD takes effect. Heparin (which has to be given by injection) is effective in controlling the rash. The two other drugs which have been reported to be helpful are tetracycline and nicotinamide.

GLUTEN-FREE DIET

Following the observation that patients with DH have an enteropathy identical to that of CD, it was shown that both the skin lesions and the enteropathy improved with gluten withdrawal from the diet[19].

There are two main points to be stressed when treating patients with DH with a GFD. First, it must be appreciated that it takes on average 6–8 months before there is any reduction of drug requirements and 24–28 months before patients no longer require any drugs for control of their rash. It must also be stressed that the response of the rash in DH depends on the strictness of the diet. It is unlikely that patients will be able to discontinue drugs unless the diet is absolutely strict. If there are occasional lapses in the diet then reduction of the dose of drugs may be obtained, but patients are unlikely to be able to discontinue drugs. If there is a regular intake of gluten, although the amount is reduced, then there is unlikely to be any reduction in the drug requirements. Because the improvement in enteropathy is more rapid than that of the skin lesions, many dermatologists and gastroenterologists did not think that a GFD was helpful in the control of the rash and discontinued it.

The second point is that only two-thirds of patients with DH show villous atrophy on intestinal biopsy (a single specimen). However, in the remaining third, although there is normal morphology of the villi, there is abnormality of the mucosa as evidenced by infiltration of the epithelium with lymphocytes and of lymphocytes and plasma cells into the sub-basement membrane region of the mucosa. The features represent so-called latent CD. Unfortunately, gastroenterologists did not accept this particular histological pattern as CD. The definition of CD until the 1990s included villous atrophy. Now it is recognized that mild or latent CD may not exhibit villous atrophy. Gastroenterologists originally considered that the one-third of DH patients not showing villous atrophy did not have a gluten-sensitivity enteropathy (CD) and thought that a GFD was not indicated. Thus, these DH patients were denied the benefit of a GFD. It has been shown that in all patients with DH the rash improves with a GFD, and there is no difference in the time it takes to clear the rash in patients with less severe features of gluten sensitivity.

As in CD, the GFD for DH must be considered as life-long treatment. It has been shown that in patients whose DH rash is controlled by a GFD even for 10 years, the eruption will recur on reintroduction of gluten, on average within 12 weeks[29].

It is important that before patients commence a GFD they are seen by a dietitian, and that the diet is supervised by the dietitian. It is also helpful for patients to join a celiac patient support group, i.e. the Celiac Society in the country in which they reside.

Advantages of a gluten-free diet

The obvious advantage of a GFD for DH patients is that eventually they will not require drugs to control their eruption. In addition, not only does the diet control the skin lesions, but it also heals the enteropathy.

One of the complications of DH and CD is the development of lymphoma. It has been shown that a GFD will protect against this complication after the diet has been taken for 5 years[30]. There are conflicting reports as to whether gluten withdrawal will prevent and/or improve autoimmune disorders associated with DH and CD[31–33].

Reasons for not taking a gluten-free diet

There are a number of reasons why DH patients do not wish to take or to persist with a GFD: (1) patients find the diet too difficult or unpalatable; (2) it is socially limiting; and (3) it is not practical, for example if they travel a great deal in their work.

Oats and a gluten-free diet

Until recently it was always advised that patients taking a GFD should avoid wheat, rye, barley and oats. This was based on challenge studies with various cereals and measuring subsequent steatorrhea and xylose absorption, but not on small-bowel biopsy. In addition, the purity of the oats was not studied. It is well known that oats are frequently contaminated with other cereals because of crop rotation by farmers and in the milling process. However, it has now been shown that pure oats are not toxic to patients with CD or DH. In addition, in patients in whom the IgA has disappeared from the skin with a long-term GFD, the IgA does not reappear with the introduction of oats to the diet. Thus, patients with CD or DH may take oats in their diet, but it must be guaranteed that the oats are pure and not contaminated by other cereals.

Long-term follow-up

Patients with DH should be kept under long-term surveillance, first because of side-effects of the drug they may be taking and second to screen them for associated disorders. Patients not taking a GFD but whose rash is controlled by drugs should be seen every 6 months and have a full blood count and biochemical screen. The latter may detect diabetes mellitus and autoimmune liver disorders. All patients, whether they are controlled by a GFD or not, should have an autoantibody screen for organ-specific antibodies. If detected, then the subjects should be screened annually for the disease(s).

In patients not taking a GFD the possibility of lymphoma should always be borne in mind when they attend for follow-up.

Patients completely controlled with a GFD should be seen yearly and screened for autoimmune disorders, as there is controversy as to whether a GFD will stop the progression to autoimmune diseases.

ASSOCIATED DISEASES

Lymphoma

There is an increased incidence of lymphoma in both CD and DH. The reported incidence has varied from 1 to 8.3%[34,35]. Originally it was reported that the lymphoma was a T-cell one arising in the small intestine. However, it has now been shown that both B-cell lymphoma and lymphoma arising at sites other than the small intestine are also increased.

A GFD is protective against the development of lymphoma in both CD and DH. If the diet has been taken for at least 5 years then the incidence of lymphoma is no higher than in the general population[30,36]. This is an important observation and should be stressed when discussing a GFD with dermatitis herpetiformis patients. The pathogenesis of lymphoma in CD and DH has not been elucidated but there are two hypotheses. The first is that there is a primary abnormality of the immune system as evidenced by splenic atrophy and small atrophic lymph nodes, and the second is chronic stimulation of the T cells in the intestine by gluten peptides. It is possible that both the abnormality of the immune system and chronic antigen stimulation of the immune system play a part in the induction of lymphoma.

Autoimmune disorders

There is a significant increase in so-called autoimmune disorders in both CD and DH. The incidence has been reported to be 19.1% in CD and 9.5% in DH. The three most commonly associated disorders in DH are thyroid disease, insulin-dependent diabetes and pernicious anemia. In one center the incidence of thyroid disease was reported as 5%, pernicious anemia 3% and insulin-dependent diabetes 2%[4]. However, there is a considerably higher incidence of the autoantibodies, thyroid being 48% and gastric parietal cell 29%. In addition, the other autoimmune disorders found in DH are myasthenia gravis, chronic active hepatitis, sclerosing cholangitis, primary biliary cirrhosis and systemic lupus erythematosus.

There are conflicting reports as to whether gluten withdrawal will prevent the development of autoantibodies and autoimmune disease. One study examined thyroid and pancreatic antibodies in CD in two groups of adolescent CD patients, one of which took a GFD and the other a normal diet. The authors reported a beneficial effect of gluten withdrawal on antibody production[32]. However, other studies have not reported a beneficial effect of gluten withdrawal on antibody production or the development of autoimmune disease[31,33].

DIFFERENTIAL DIAGNOSIS

There are a number of very itchy conditions which may be difficult to distinguish from DH on clinical grounds. However, with the advent of the criterion for DH being IgA in uninvolved skin of DH patients, it is now very easy to distinguish other itchy eruptions from DH.

Eczema

Endogenous eczemas may present with severe irritating eruptions, and if symmetrical and involving the extensor forearms and buttocks may be confused with DH. Excoriations are common in both conditions and may be the predominant sign. Further confusion may arise as the irritation associated with eczema may also respond to dapsone.

Scabies

Scabies is a very itchy condition, and the buttocks are a common site of involvement. There are three types of skin lesion in scabies. First, 'burrows' may occur on the hands and wrists. The second are large 0.5–1.0-cm red papules on the buttocks, around the axillae and on the genitalia in males. The latter are pathognomonic. Third, there may be a widespread eruption on the trunk and limbs consisting mainly of small papules (less than 0.5 cm).

The diagnosis of scabies can be substantiated by finding the above types and sites of lesions. Also, a positive family history is helpful in establishing the diagnosis.

Papular urticaria (insect bites)

In some patients this may be a chronic eruption if the source of the insect is in the home or work place. The lesions may be associated with blisters and be persistent. However, the lesions are usually not symmetrical and do not show a predilection for the extensor forearms and buttocks.

Neurotic excoriations

As the name implies, the predominant skin lesion is an excoriation which presents as scabs and may be linear. The patient describes their eruption as intensely irritating. The distribution of the eruption is often determined by the ease with which the skin can be reached, e.g. extensor forearms, outer legs, upper and lower back, with sparing of the upper back between the posterior shoulders and mid-back. No other skin lesions are seen and the patient admits to scratching.

Prurigo nodularis

This condition is also associated with irritation, but the characteristic lesion is an excoriated nodule (0.5–1.0 cm). The lesions may be widespread, but again are common in the sites which are easy for the patient to scratch, i.e. outer arms, lateral aspect of legs, buttocks and upper back.

It is thought by some that patients who present with prurigo nodularis are basically atopic.

Linear IgA disease

Linear IgA disease (LAD) is another 'blistering disorder' with IgA in the skin. However, in LAD the IgA is found in a homogeneous band along the line of the basement membrane. It presents with small blisters arranged at the periphery of a discoid plaque, the so-called 'crown of jewels'. Its sites of predilection are the axillae and groins, and in children the pubic area. However, it may be widespread and become generalized. Like DH, LAD responds to dapsone, and the diagnosis has to be made by determining the pattern of IgA deposition using immunofluorescent tests.

3 Pemphigus

The name pemphigus is derived from the Greek word 'pemphix', or blister. There are two main subdivisions of pemphigus based on clinical and histological features, namely pemphigus vulgaris (PV) and pemphigus foliaceus (PF). In both types of pemphigus the primary site of pathology is the epidermis. In PV it is the lower, whilst in PF it is the upper epidermis, just below the stratum corneum.

EPIDEMIOLOGY

Pemphigus is a rare disease, the overall incidence being estimated as 0.75–5.0 per million per year. PV is more common than PF in the Western world, approximately 3 : 1.

PV is most common in the Middle East (Jews and Muslims) and in the Indian subcontinent, Malaysia and China. In the West it is more common in Ashkenazi Jews than in the remainder of the Caucasian population[37]. PF is more prevalent in Africa[38], whilst so-called endemic PF is seen in Brazil and is sometimes referred to as Brazilian pemphigus or 'fogo selvagem' (wild fire).

ETIOLOGY

Genetic factors

PV is linked to certain human leukocyte antigen (HLA) alleles. Thus, HLA-DRBI*0402 is associated with the disease in Ashkanazi Jews[39] and DRBI*1401/04 and DQBI*0503 in non-Jewish patients of European or Asian descent[40]. PF is associated with HLA-DRBI*0102 and 0404. The susceptibility genes in endemic or Brazilian pemphigus are HLA-DRBI*0102, 0404, 1402 and 1406*[41]. Although the clinical appearances of PF and Brazilian pemphigus are the same, in the latter the age group affected is considerably younger, the disease being seen in children and young adults.

Apart from Brazilian pemphigus, it is uncommon to find PV and PF in family members of the affected individuals, although it has been claimed that there is a higher incidence of other autoimmune disorders, e.g. myasthenia gravis, lupus erythematosus and thymoma. However, there is no associated increase of autoimmune disorders associated with the haplotype B8/DR3/DQ1, i.e. thyroid disease, insulin-dependent disorders and pernicious anemia.

Environmental factors

It is possible that certain micro-organisms may trigger pemphigus, as has been suggested for other autoimmune disorders. Viral DNA (herpes simplex, Epstein–Barr and herpes viruses 6 and 8) has been detected in some skin biopsies and blood from some PV patients. PF is more common than PV in Africa, and this is thought to be perhaps related to micro-organisms possibly transmitted by insect bites.

In endemic Brazilian pemphigus it has been found that the disorder is more common in rural areas and at the end of the rainy season when insects are most abundant. Bites from the insect 'black fly' are a risk factor for the disease, and it is possible that the 'bite' contains substances which are antigenic, or that the fly transmits an infectious agent which acts as a trigger.

PATHOLOGY

The characteristic features of pemphigus are an intraepidermal blister and acantholytic cells. In PV the blister occurs in the lower epidermis, just above the basal cells (Figure 3.1), whilst in PF the blister is seen in the upper epidermis below the stratum corneum. The earliest change in PV is intercellular edema with loss of intercellular attachments. In PV the suprabasal cells separate from the basal cells, which remain attached to the basement membrane but detach from each other and stand like a row of 'tombstones'.

Acantholysis is the term given to separation of the epidermal cells from each other. The cells are found floating in the blister fluid, and have lost their spinous processes and appear as dark, rounded cells. The intracellular cytokeratin tonofilaments retract around the nucleus, and the desmosomal plaques disappear. Eosinophils are sometimes seen infiltrating the epidermis. In the dermis there is an inflammatory cell infiltrate of lymphocytes and histiocytes.

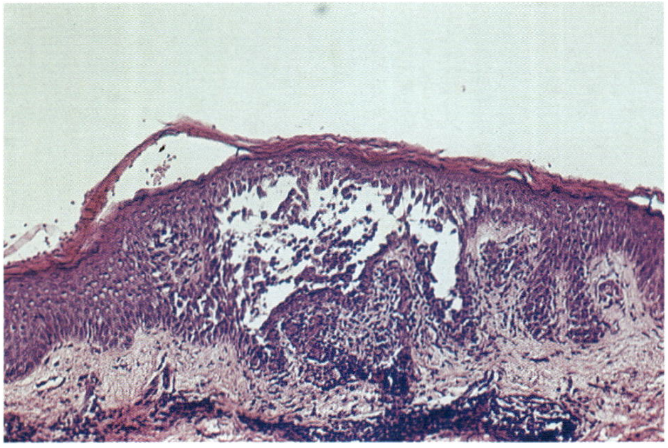

Figure 3.1 Pemphigus vulgaris intraepidermal blister with acantholytic cells in the blister. The split in the epidermis has occurred in the lower part just above the basement membrane

PATHOGENESIS

The primary pathological event in pemphigus is the loss of adhesion of the epidermal cells. The attachment of epidermal cells is mainly through the desmosomes, and to a lesser extent by so-called 'tight' or 'adherence' junctions. The desmosome is made up of structures called cadherins which are divided into desmogleins and desmocollins. These structures have an intracellular, a transmembrane and an extracellular component. Intracellularly they are attached to the keratin cytoskeleton and extracellularly to that of another cell forming the desmosome (Figure 3.2). Desmogleins are subdivided into desmogleins 1, 2 and 3 and are intracellular components of the desmosome (Figure 3.2). Desmoglein 3 is expressed only in the basal and suprabasal layers of the epidermis, whereas desmoglein 1 is expressed throughout the epidermis but mainly in the upper layers. In mucosae, desmoglein 3 is strongly expressed throughout the epithelium and desmoglein 1 only weakly.

Desmoglein 3 has been called the PV antigen and desmoglein 1 the PF antigen. However, there is some

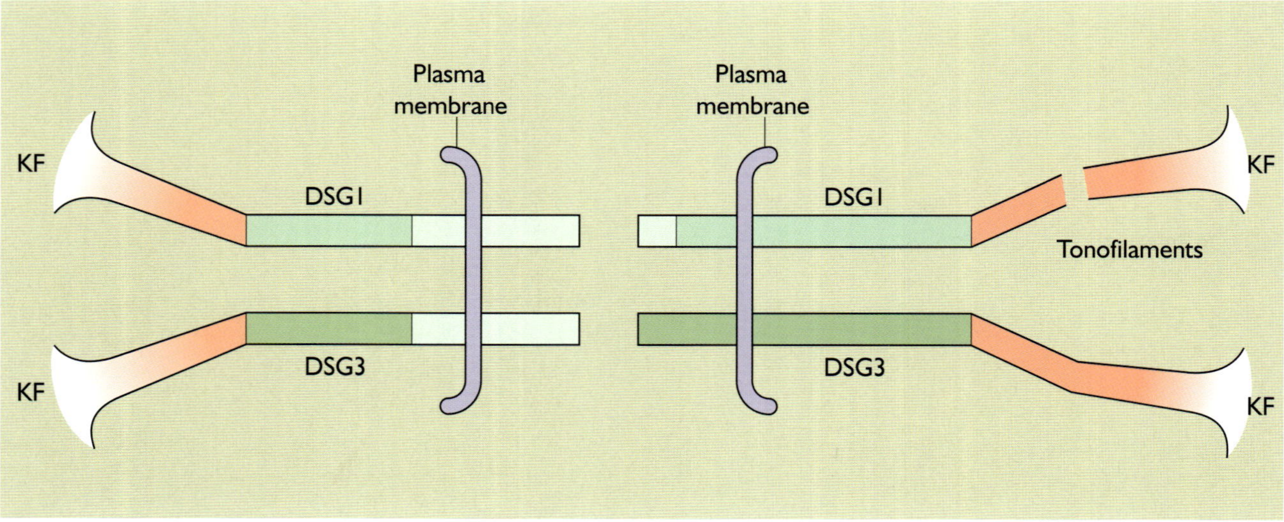

Figure 3.2 Desmosome: intercellular connection. DSG1, desmoglein 1; DSG3, desmoglein 3; KF, keratin filament

overlap between the two desmogleins, and where both desmogleins are expressed one molecule is able to compensate for loss of function of the other (the so-called compensatory theory).

In pemphigus, desmoglein antibodies are found both fixed to the skin and circulating in the blood. These antibodies have been termed intercellular, as their localization on direct microscopy reflects this pattern. However, the antibodies are probably binding to cell surface antigens. Circulating antibodies are found in approximately 80% of patients, and the titer correlates with the severity of the disease. Antibodies are found in the skin in 95–100% of patients. The antibodies are immunoglobulin G (IgG), but occasionally IgA and IgM and C3 complement may be deposited at the same sites.

The antibodies in pemphigus are considered to be pathogenic. They have been shown to induce features of pemphigus on organ culture of human skin, and when passively administered to neonatal mice. The lesions in mice can be inhibited by absorbing out the antibodies to desmogleins 1 and 3 from pemphigus sera. In addition, it has been observed in pregnant patients with pemphigus that placental transfer of maternal autoantibodies occurs, with the development of skin lesions in newborn babies.

Whether the antibodies actually cause the lesions is related to the IgG subclass. IgG1 antibodies are present in individuals without skin lesions, but IgG4 antibodies are invariably present in patients with active disease.

There has been an attempt to correlate the site of the lesions with the autoantibodies: oral lesions are more common in patients with only desmoglein 3 antibodies, oral and other mucosal lesions are found only if antibodies are present to both desmoglein 1 and desmoglein 3, and skin lesions without oral lesions are present only with desmoglein 1. The desmoglein compensatory theory has also been invoked to explain this apparent relationship[42]. According to this theory, oral lesions are seen only in PV because desmoglein 3 antibodies are present, and only desmoglein 3 is present in the oral mucosa. However, this does not explain why lesions do not occur in all layers of the oral mucosa, since there is no desmoglein 1 to compensate for the inactivation of desmoglein 3. Furthermore, the theory does not explain why antibodies to both desmoglein 3 and desmoglein 1 are necessary for lesions to appear on the skin, and yet the site of pathology is the lower epidermis where there is no desmoglein 1 and where antibodies to desmoglein 1 have no effect.

Why patients with pemphigus develop antibodies in the first place is not known, but environmental factors may be important in their initiation.

CLINICAL FEATURES

Pemphigus vulgaris

This type of pemphigus affects the sexes equally and most commonly presents in middle age, although it may present earlier in subjects from the Indian subcontinent, the Middle East and North Africa. Mucosal lesions are common in PV, and 50% of patients present with oral lesions. These lesions may precede skin lesions by months, and may be the only manifestation of the disease. The lesions in the mouth usually present as painful ulcers, as the blisters that form soon rupture due to trauma from eating. The superficial ulcers or erosions are usually multiple and have a red base and irregular edge (Figure 3.3). The mucosa around the ulcers has a normal appearance. The lesions are persistent and rarely heal. There is a predilection for buccal (Figure 3.4), labial (Figure 3.5), tongue (Figure 3.6) and palatal mucosae (Figure 3.3). The lips themselves are also affected (Figure 3.7).

Other mucosal sites include the pharynx, larynx, nose, upper esophagus, vulva, urethra, cervix and conjunctiva. Involvement of the pharynx and esophagus presents with dysphagia, the larynx as hoarseness and nasal mucosa as congestion and/or bloody discharge.

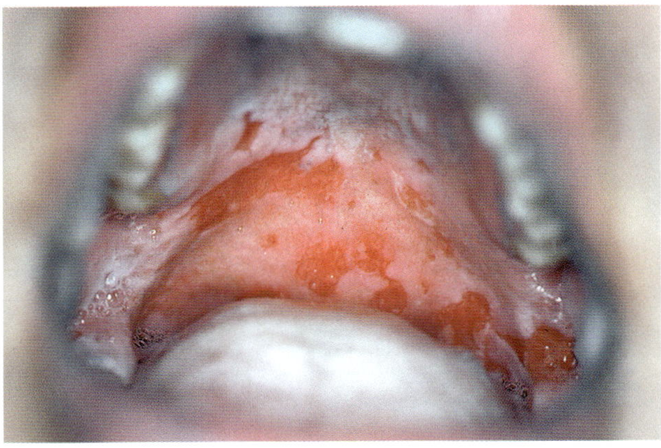

Figure 3.3 Multiple red-based ulcers on the palate in pemphigus vulgaris

The sites of predilection for the skin lesions are the scalp, face (Figure 3.8) and upper trunk (Figures 3.9 and 3.10), although other sites may also be involved and the eruption may become generalized in severe disease (Figure 3.11). It should be remembered that PV may begin with skin and not mucosal lesions. Although mucosal lesions are common, none may occur.

The initial skin lesion is a flaccid bulla (Figure 3.12) filled with a clear fluid, but may become opaque with a yellow fluid due to polymorphonuclear cells (Figure 3.12). As the roof of the blister is thin in pemphigus it soon ruptures, and superficial erosions result (Figures 3.9–3.12). The erosions may extend and become large. Crusting of the erosions is common (Figures 3.13 and 3.14). It must be stressed that although pemphigus is one of the 'blistering diseases', none may be seen when the patient presents for the first time. Superficial erosions and crusted lesions are the common forms of presentation (Figures 3.8–3.15).

As the skin around the bulla is likely to be involved, it is sometimes possible by applying gentle lateral pressure with a finger to produce an erosion of the surrounding skin. This is termed the Nikolsky sign.

PV lesions heal without scarring, but altered pigmentation and (Figure 3.16) milia may occur.

If left untreated, large erosions will form, which frequently become infected, and fluid loss, as with burns, will result in metabolic disturbance.

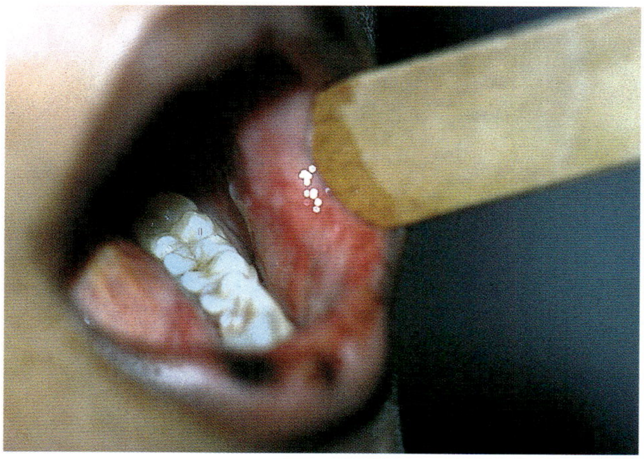

Figure 3.4 Superficial ulcers on the buccal mucosa in pemphigus vulgaris

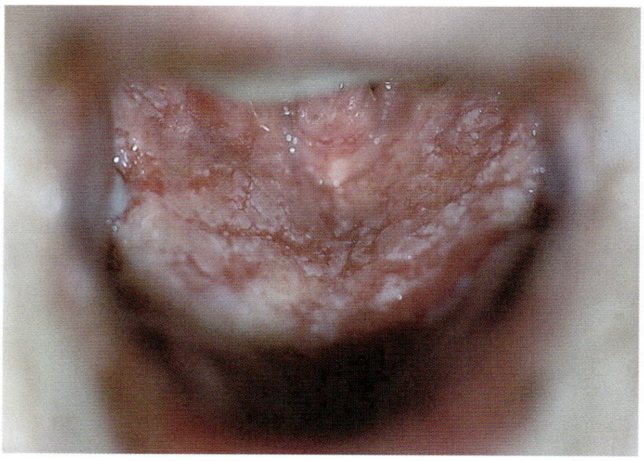

Figure 3.6 Erosions on the tongue, with secondary *Candida albicans* infection related to immunosuppressive treatment

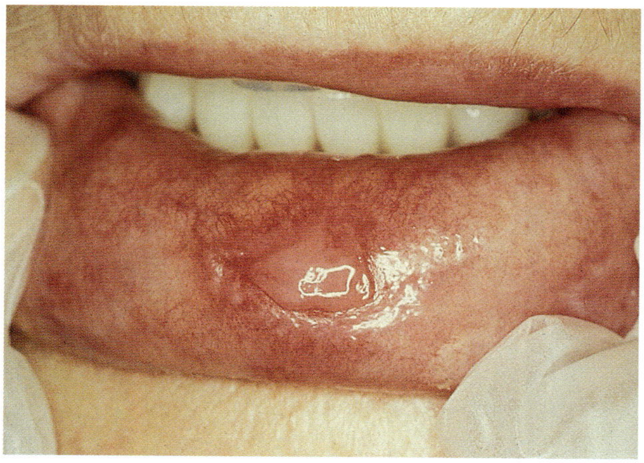

Figure 3.5 Erosions on the mucosal surface of the lower lip

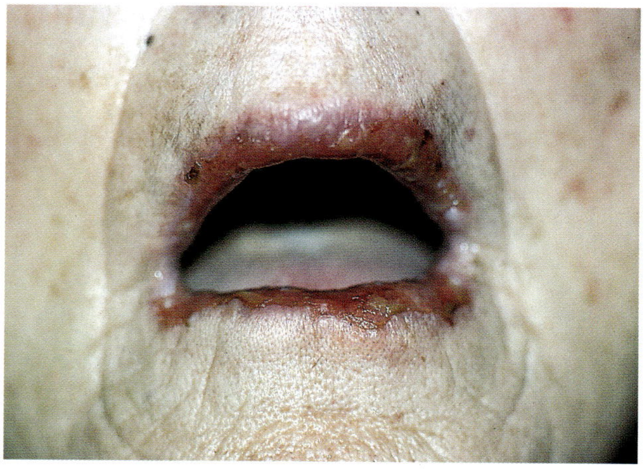

Figure 3.7 Erosions and crusts on the lips

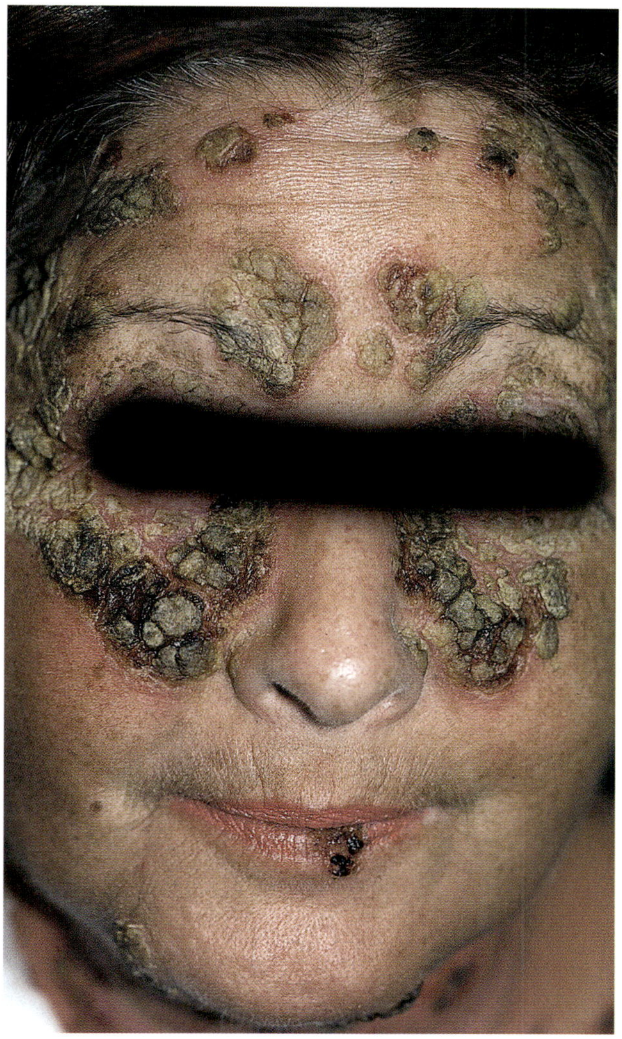

Figure 3.8 Crusted lesions on the face in pemphigus vulgaris

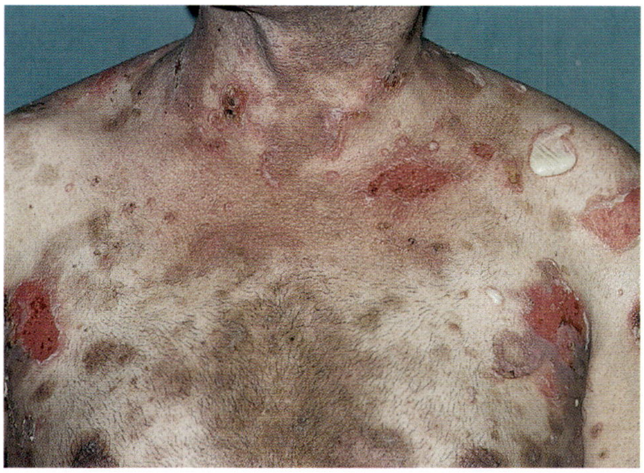

Figure 3.9 Large erosions and older hyperpigmented healing lesions on the upper trunk, a common site for pemphigus vulgaris

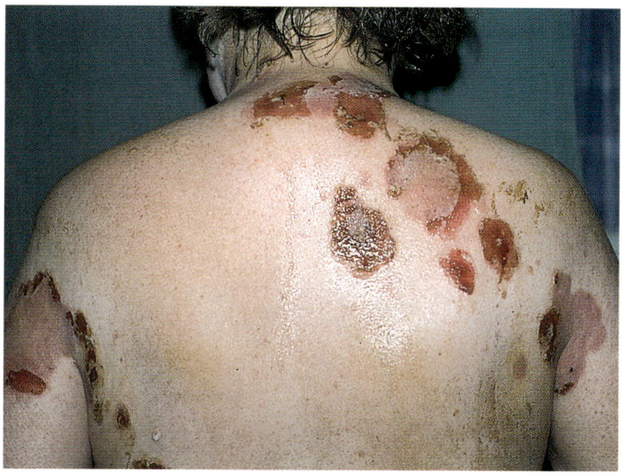

Figure 3.10 Large erosions on the upper back in pemphigus vulgaris

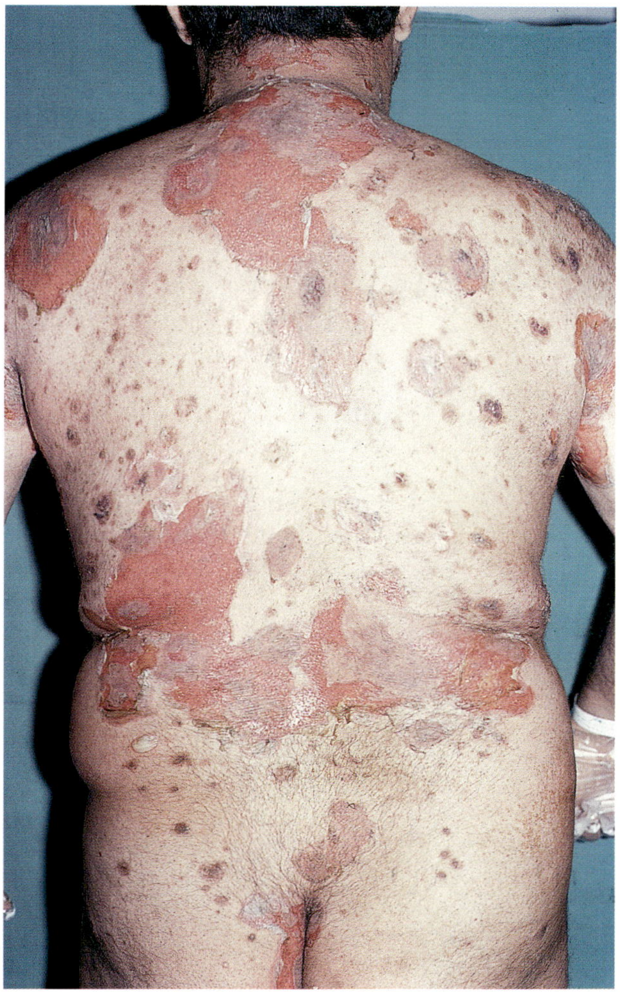

Figure 3.11 Widespread involvement on the trunk in pemphigus vulgaris

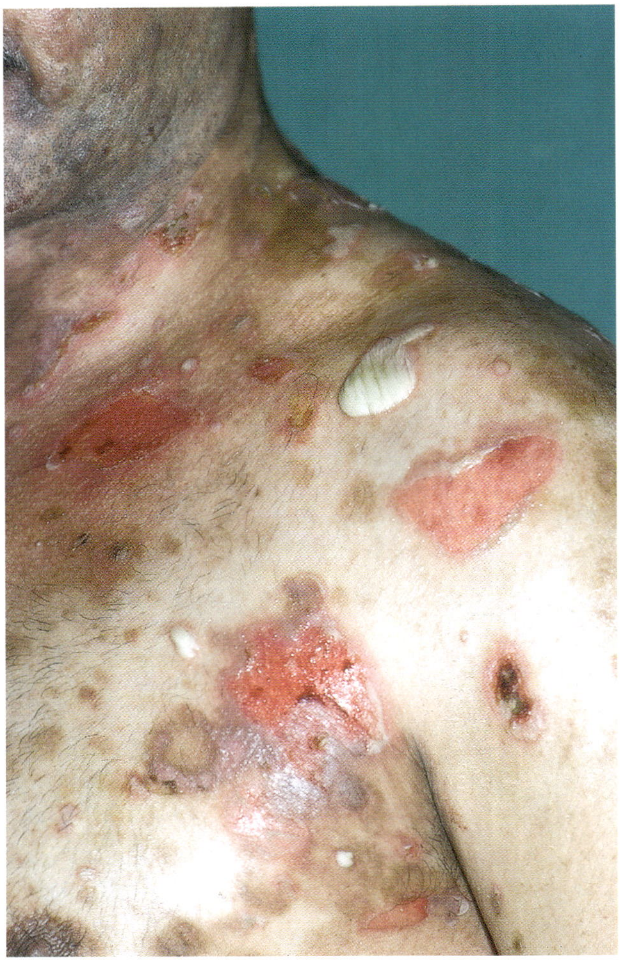

Figure 3.12 Flaccid blisters and erosions in pemphigus

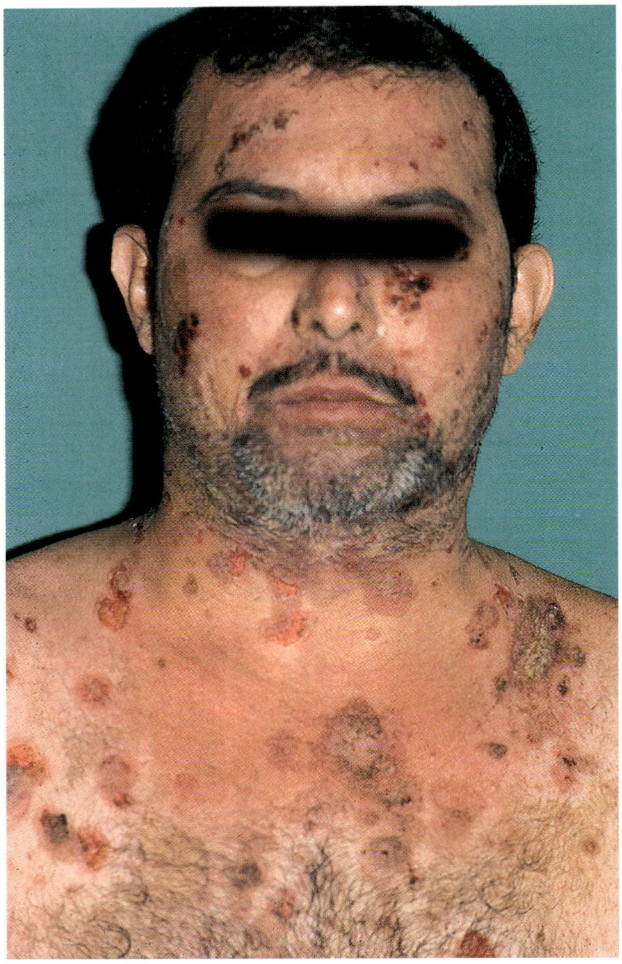

Figure 3.14 Crusted lesions on the face and upper trunk in pemphigus vulgaris

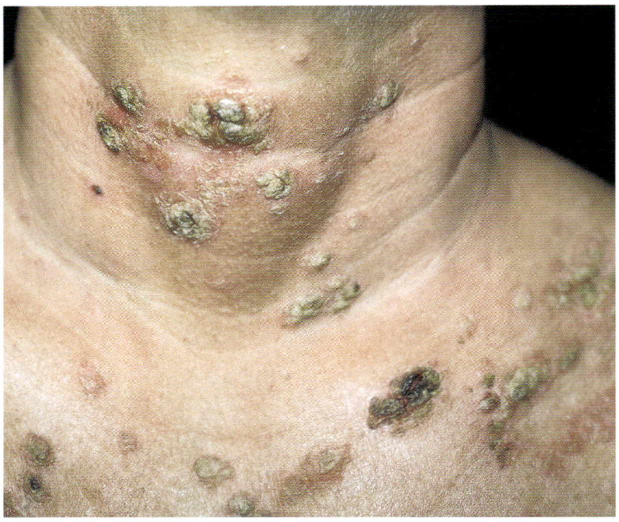

Figure 3.13 Thick crusted lesions in pemphigus

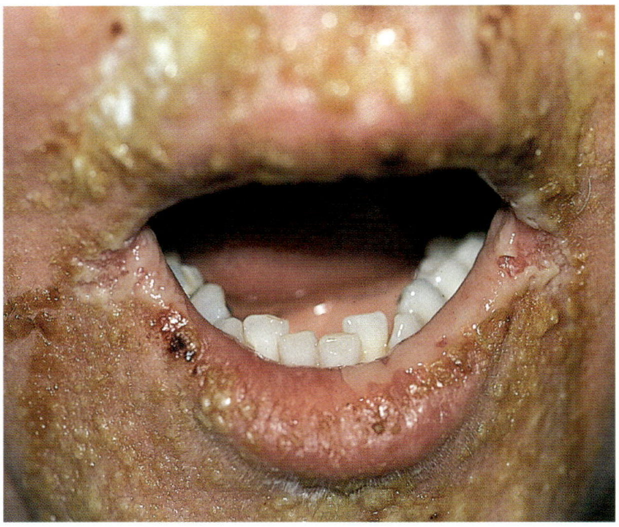

Figure 3.15 Crusting on the lips and around the mouth in pemphigus vulgaris

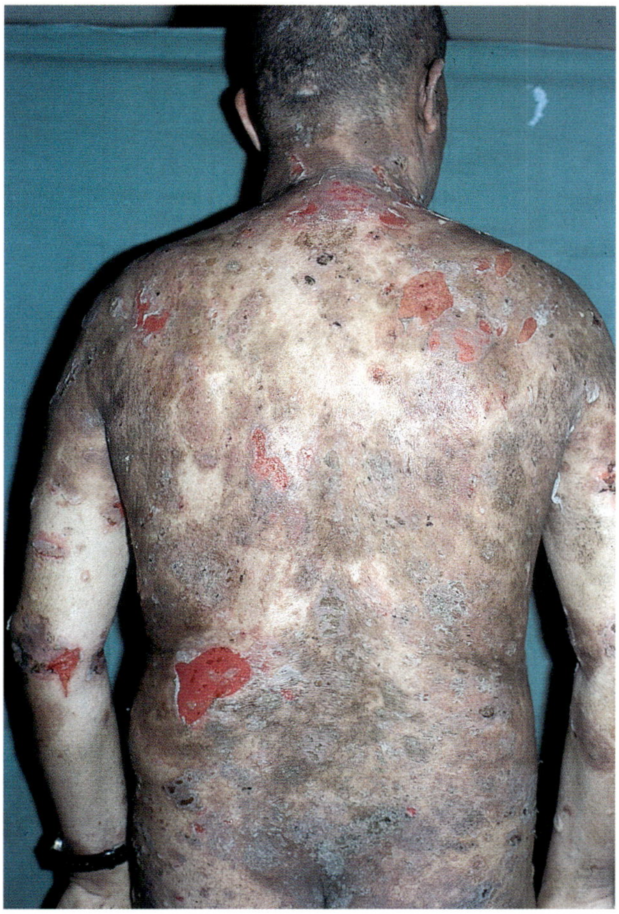

Figure 3.16 Hyperpigmentation after healing of pemphigus lesions

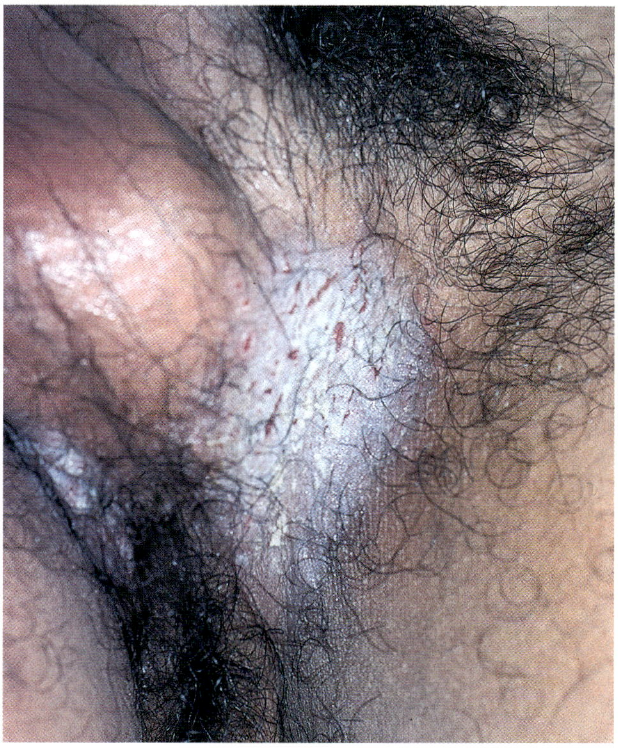

Figure 3.17 Pemphigus vegetans in the groin

Pemphigus vegetans is a variant of PV in which healing of the lesions is associated with vegetating proliferation of the epidermis. The common sites for this type of the disease are the intertriginous areas, i.e. the groins (Figure 3.17), axillae and submammary regions. Secondary infection is common and crusting may occur.

SUPERFICIAL PEMPHIGUS

There are subtypes of superficial pemphigus: pemphigus foliaceus, pemphigus erythematosus and endemic (Brazilian) pemphigus.

Pemphigus foliaceus

Pemphigus foliaceus (PF) is less common than PV. It affects the sexes equally and usually presents in middle age. The lesions occur mainly on the scalp, face (Figure 3.18) and upper trunk (Figures 3.19 and

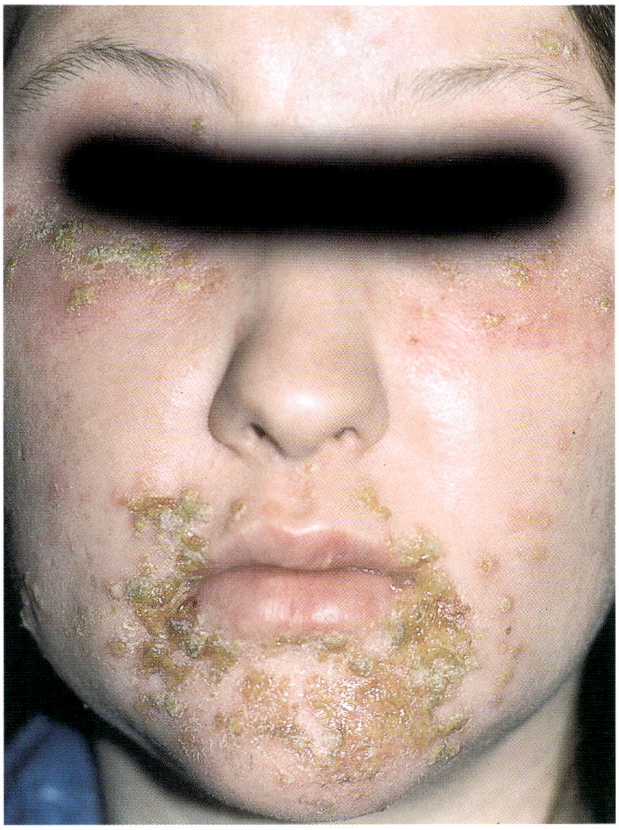

Figure 3.18 Red superficial scaly and crusted patches in pemphigus foliaceus

3.20). As the site of pathology is the upper epidermis just below the stratum corneum, there is too little tissue to trap fluid and form a blister. The lesions arise from normal-looking skin as red crusted patches (Figure 3.19). The crusts can easily be removed, leaving superficial erosions (Figure 3.20). Untreated, the lesions do not heal and become confluent, and may involve all the skin to give a similar appearance to erythroderma from eczema and/or psoriasis. Unlike PV, oral lesions rarely occur.

Pemphigus erythematosus

Pemphigus erythematosus is a variant of PF, and presents as red scaly/crusted lesions on the nose and cheeks (Figure 3.21) in the so-called butterfly distribution. Lesions on the trunk may occur, and have a similar appearance to PF (Figure 3.22).

The name pemphigus erythematosus is derived from the fact that the distribution of the rash is that of systemic lupus erythematosus. In addition, patients have immunoglobulin deposits with features of both diseases, i.e. there is IgG intercellular deposition and granular deposits of IgG at the basement membrane region. It is rare for patients to progress to systemic lupus erythematosus and it has been suggested that the immunoglobulin deposits at the basement membrane are not related to lupus erythematosus but occur due to chronic exposure to sunlight, and this finding is well recognized.

Endemic pemphigus foliaceus

This has been reported in Brazil, Peru, El Salvador and Colombia.

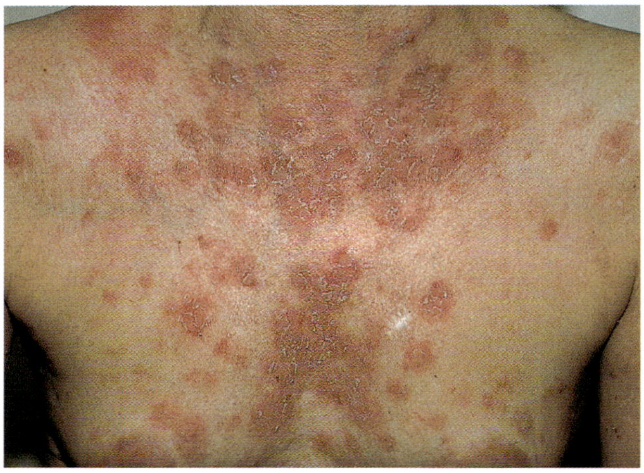

Figure 3.19 Discrete red scaly and slightly crusted lesions in pemphigus foliaceus

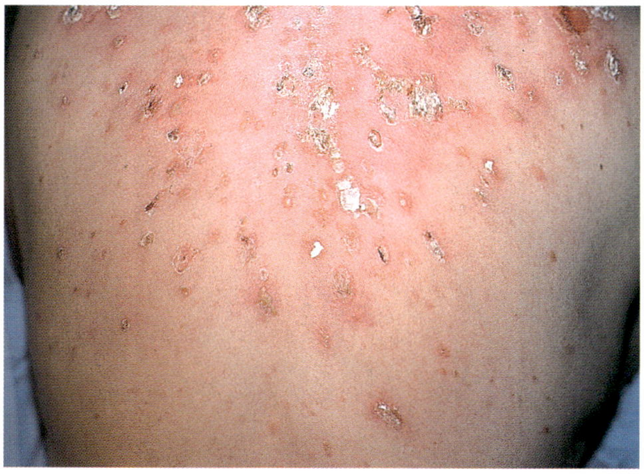

Figure 3.20 Red superficial scaly patches on the back in pemphigus foliaceus. In one lesion on the right upper back crusts have been removed to reveal a superficial erosion

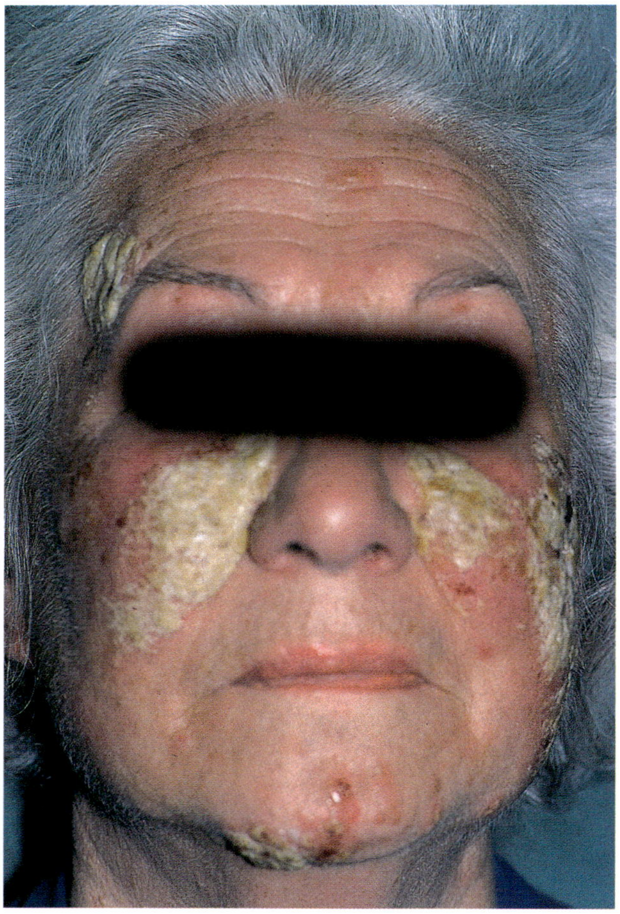

Figure 3.21 Red scaly crusted lesions on the cheeks in pemphigus erythematosus

Endemic PF usually occurs in children and young adults, unlike other forms of pemphigus which are usually seen in middle age.

The lesions first appear on the head and neck, and may subsequently spread to involve the trunk and limbs. Although the site of pathology is the upper epidermis, flaccid bullae occur which rupture quickly, giving rise to erosions. The burnt appearance and burning sensation have given rise to the name fogo selvagem (Portuguese for 'wild fire'). If the disease becomes extensive, generalized erythroderma may occur.

Antibodies to desmoglein 1 are the main antibodies found in affected individuals.

DRUG-INDUCED PEMPHIGUS

Drugs containing a sulfhydryl group (thiol drugs) such as penicillamine and captopril are the drugs most commonly associated with the induction of pemphigus. Pemphigus has also been attributed to other angiotensin-converting enzyme inhibitors, e.g. enalapril, ramipril and fosinopril, as well as other drugs, including nifedipine and the antibiotic rifampicin, penicillins and cephalosporins. Interferons have also been reported to induce pemphigus.

The type of pemphigus most commonly seen with drugs is pemphigus foliaceus or erythematosus. The same antibodies are present as occur in spontaneous forms of the disease. It has been reported that 50% of patients with permphigus due to the thiol drugs will remit spontaneously when the drugs are discontinued. Spontaneous remission is less common with non-thiol drugs.

INVESTIGATIONS

Immunological

Direct immunofluorescence of perilesional skin is the most reliable test for establishing the diagnosis. IgG deposits on the surface of the keratinocytes giving a 'crazy pavement' appearance are diagnostic of pemphigus (Figure 3.23). Antibodies detected by indirect immunofluorescence are present in approximately 80% of patients.

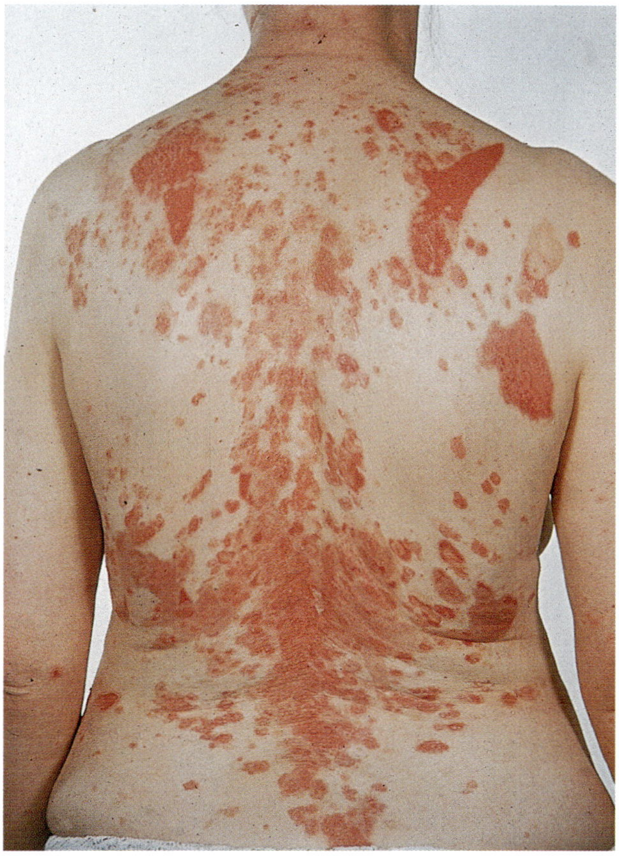

Figure 3.22 Superficial red slightly scaly patches on the back in pemphigus erythematosus

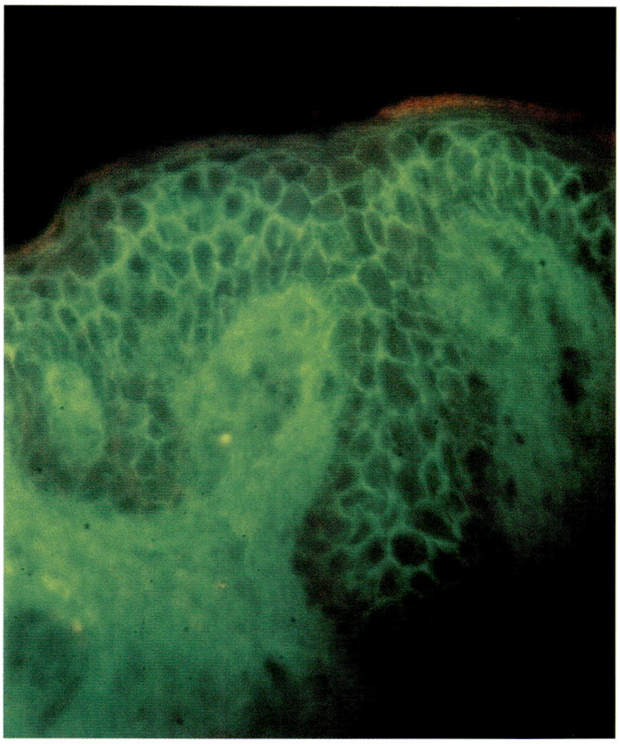

Figure 3.23 Immunoglobulin G (IgG) deposition on the surface of keratinocytes in pemphigus

Histology

The earliest feature is intercellular edema and loss of intercellular attachments. In PV, the suprabasal cells separate from the basal cells, which remain attached to the basement membrane. A fluid-filled cavity forms within which acantholytic cells are seen.

Investigations prior to treatment

As current treatment involves large doses of systemic corticosteroids and immunosuppressive drugs, it is important to screen patients for any underlying disorders. A full blood count and biochemical screen are mandatory. The latter should include liver function tests, creatinine, glucose and lipids. A chest radiograph and tuberculin test to exclude tuberculosis should be performed. Bone densitometry should be carried out, as osteoporosis is likely with high-dose and long-term steroids.

TREATMENT

This tends to be similar, irrespective of the type of pemphigus. The dose of drug will depend on the severity of the disease. The aim of treatment is to clear the lesions as quickly as possible and then gradually reduce the drug dosage to a level where no or very few new lesions appear. Systemic corticosteroids are the basis of treatment and other therapeutic modalities are used in an attempt to lessen the dose of steroids required.

Systemic corticosteroids

The initial dose of prednisolone will depend on the extent and severity of the mucosal and/or skin lesions. For severe disease, an initial dose of 120 mg daily is usually required. If after 2 weeks there is no significant improvement and new lesions are still appearing, then an increase in the dose of prednisolone can be given or alternative measures employed. If the dose of prednisolone is to be increased this should be done by 50%, i.e. to 180 mg daily, and if improvement still fails to occur after a further 2 weeks then the dose may be increased to 240 mg daily. However, if this dose is maintained for any length of time then considerable morbidity will ensue. The option is to use alternative measures (see below) and not raise the dose of prednisolone above 120 mg daily.

If the disease is mild, involving only a relatively small area of body surface, i.e. < 5%, then the initial dose may be prednisolone 60 mg daily.

Gradual reduction of the dose (i.e. 10%) of prednisolone should be attempted once the disease is under control. The speed of reduction will depend on the initial severity and whether new lesions are appearing. If no new lesions appear, the dose can be reduced by 10% every 2 weeks. The maintenance dose of prednisolone varies between patients and the rule is the lower the better, if possible below 20 mg daily. It should be stressed that further gradual reduction in dosage should be attempted if patients are in remission. It is possible to discontinue systemic steroids when a permanent remission occurs. Side-effects from systemic steroids include hypertension, diabetes mellitus, osteoporosis, upper gastrointestinal ulceration and bleeding, skeletal myopathy, cataract, weight gain, insomnia, confusional states, mania, hypokalemia and thinning of the skin.

Topical corticosteroids

These play only a small part in the management of pemphigus. Very potent (group IV) topical corticosteroids are sometimes helpful in mild pemphigus foliaceus.

Pulse therapy

Pulse therapy with intravenous methylprednisolone has been recommended for severe disease not responding to other measures. The dose is 1 g per day for 5 days. Apart from the increased risk of side-effects described above for systemic steroids, there is an additional risk of rupture of the chordae tendinae with pulse therapy.

Plasmapheresis

Plasmaphoresis can be used if patients fail to respond to a high dose of prednisolone, i.e. 120 mg or more daily. The rationale for plasmapheresis is that it physically removes the pathogenic antibodies. Treatment is performed three times in a week. Patients should in addition be given cyclophosphamide to stop a rebound in antibody production.

The main side-effect of plasmapheresis is infection, and this is a serious problem in patients taking high-dose systemic steroids and cyclophosphamide.

Intravenous immunoglobulin

Intravenous immunoglobulin (IVIg) is replacing plasmapheresis as a safer option for patients not responding to high-dose systemic steroids. IVIg has been reported to be effective in many autoimmune disorders with circulating antibodies. In pemphigus it has been shown that the antibodies fall rapidly, i.e. within 1–2 weeks. The decrease is selective as total concentrations of IgG increase. It has been proposed that IVIg rapidly increases the catabolism of immunoglobulins due to the pronounced increase in total concentration of immunoglobulin molecules from the infusion. This means that the pemphigus antibodies are selectively decreased as the concentration of other antibodies is replaced by those in the administered immunoglobulin[42].

Steroid-sparing drugs

Because of the relatively high doses and long-term treatment with such doses of systemic steroids in pemphigus, other drugs are used in an attempt to lower the dose of steroids required for control of the disease. There is a 'delayed phase' of approximately 6 weeks before these other drugs produce a clinical effect, and it has been advocated that they are started together with the systemic steroids.

Azathioprine

Azathioprine interferes with DNA synthesis and will therefore affect the proliferation of T and B lymphocytes. The dose in pemphigus is 1–2 mg/kg/day. Prior to commencing azathioprine it is important to measure serum thiopurine methyl transferase, for if this enzyme is low there will be an increase in the incidence and severity of side-effects. As clinical improvement occurs, it is possible to reduce the dose in addition to reducing the dose of corticosteroids.

Side-effects of azathioprine include bone marrow suppression, hepatotoxicity and immuno suppression. The last may lead to an increased risk of infection, and in the long term to malignancies, particularly skin cancer and lymphoma.

Mycophenolate mofetil

Mycophenolate mofetil (MMF) is a prodrug, and is hydrolyzed to mycophenolic acid (MPA). MPA is a selective, uncompetitive and reversible inhibitor of monophosphate dehydrogenase, an important enzyme in the *de novo* pathway of guanine nucleotide synthesis. B and T lymphocytes are dependent on this pathway for cell proliferation, and thus antibody production is suppressed. The dose of MMF is 1 g twice daily, and this can be increased to 1.5 g twice daily if necessary.

Side-effects of MMF are gastrointestinal (diarrhea, nausea and vomiting) and hematological (suppression of the bone marrow, particularly leukopenia). There is an increased risk of infection with cytomegalic virus and malignancies if taken long term.

Methotrexate

Methotrexate is not generally advocated for use combined with high-dose corticosteroids because of the risk of severe infection. However, occasionally it has been found that methotrexate alone can control pemphigus once the disease has been brought under partial control with large doses of corticosteroids. Methotrexate inhibits DNA synthesis and thus proliferation of T lymphocytes.

Side-effects include hepatotoxicity and bone marrow suppression. An increase in atherosclerosis has been suggested because of increased levels of homocysteine when taking methotrexate, and this can been countered by taking folic acid.

The dose of methotrexate, if taken with systemic steroids, should be kept moderately low, i.e. 10–15 mg weekly.

Cyclosporine

Cyclosporine is a calcineuron inhibitor, and blocks the production of cytokines by T lymphocytes. The dose should not exceed 5 mg/kg/day. Side-effects are hypertension and nephrotoxicity.

Rituximab

Rituximab is an anti-CD20 monoclonal antibody against B cells. The rationale for its use is that it will suppress antibody production. A recent report of five patients with pemphigus, four with vulgaris and one with foliaceus, showed significant improvement of their disease which correlated with a fall in desmoglein 1 and 3 antibodies[43].

Dapsone

Dapsone has been claimed to have some success in mild PV and PF. Side-effects include hemolysis, depression, headache and entrapment neuropathy.

Tetracyclines

Tetracyclines have been shown to be helpful when combined with systemic steroids.

Topical preparations for the oral mucosa

Apart from systemic drugs which are required for oral pemphigus, cyclosporine and Betnesol® mouthwashes have been shown to be helpful.

NATURAL HISTORY AND PROGNOSIS

The prognosis in PV is worse than in PF. In PV, patients with the most severe forms of the disease will die within a year without treatment. If the disease is mild then the prognosis is better, and drug-induced or spontaneous remission may occur even within a few months of onset. The advent of systemic steroids in the 1950s altered the prognosis. The mortality rate for PV is now less than 10%, and most patients succumb to the side-effects of treatment rather than the disease *per se*. The activity of PV tends to wane after 2 years, and drug requirements decrease. PV patients with severe disease will often require indefinite treatment, but in others remission will occur and these patients no longer require treatment. It has been estimated that the average duration of treatment for all patients with PV is approximately 7 years.

PF has a better prognosis than PV. Untreated, it runs a protracted course over many years. PF responds better to treatment than PV and requires a lower dose of systemic steroids for control.

DIFFERENTIAL DIAGNOSIS

PV has to be distinguished from the other bullous disorders including pemphigoid, linear IgA disease, dermatitis herpetiformis and erythema multiforme. However, with the advent of direct and indirect immunofluorescent studies it is now easier to differentiate the various bullous disorders.

Pemphigoid

This tends to occur in an older age group. The lesions occur most commonly on the limbs, and the blisters are often situated on urticarial plaques, unlike pemphigus. In addition, blisters in pemphigoid, being subepidermal, are tense and do not rupture so easily.

Dermatitis herpetiformis

The lesions in dermatitis herpetiformis (DH) characteristically occur on the elbows, buttocks and knees, which are uncommon sites for pemphigus. The lesions of DH tend to be intensely irritating, and may present as scabs due to scratching. Erosions and crusted lesions are rare in DH.

Linear IgA disease

This dermatosis often involves the groins and axillae and has to be distinguished from pemphigus vegetans. However, blisters are not usually present in the latter, but are in linear IgA disease (LAD). The blisters in LAD are tense as they are subepidermal, and are often found in an annular configuration, unlike pemphigus.

Erythema multiforme

Classic erythema multiforme will have target lesions on the hands. On the trunk and limbs the lesions tend to occur on an urticarial base. Erythema multiforme may show oral lesions, and immunofluorescent studies may have to be performed to distinguish between pemphigus and erythema multiforme.

Lupus erythematosus

Pemphigus erythematosus has to be distinguished from lupus erythematosus. Immunofluorescent studies of the skin and the detection of antinuclear antibodies in lupus erythematosus will allow the correct diagnosis to be made.

Seborrheic eczema

This may resemble pemphigus foliaceus as both affect similar areas on the face and trunk. Both are chronic disorders, and may have to be distinguished by immunofluorescent studies.

Staphylococcal disorders

Widespread impetigo with crusting and erosions may resemble pemphigus, particularly if the face is involved. Swabs taken for bacteriology and a rapid response to antibiotics should distinguish the two diseases.

Staphylococcal scalded-skin syndrome may present with blisters and widespread erosions. The sudden onset of this disorder helps to distinguish it from pemphigus, which often has a slow, insidious onset.

Drug eruptions

Bullous drug eruptions are of sudden onset and widespread. A detailed history of drug intake (essential in all patients) may help in the diagnosis.

Oral lesions

The disorders which have to be distinguished from pemphigus include viral infections, benign mucous membrane pemphigoid, linear IgA disease, chronic aphthous ulcers, Stevens–Johnson syndrome and Behçet's disease.

Primary herpes simplex tends to be of sudden onset and self-limiting. Mucous membrane pemphigoid is also persistent and painful, although the gums are frequently affected, unlike pemphigus. Linear IgA disease may affect the mucous membranes and the skin as in pemphigus. Immunofluorescent studies will give the correct diagnosis. Chronic aphthosis of the mouth presents with painful ulcers often on a yellow base, which are often self-limiting but at times become a chronic problem. Steven–Johnson syndrome has erythema multiforme lesions on the limbs and trunk, the eyes and genitalia are involved and the disease is of sudden onset.

PARANEOPLASTIC PEMPHIGUS

The exact nosology of so-called paraneoplastic pemphigus (PNP) is uncertain. It has been termed pemphigus, because on histology there is suprabasal clefting and acantholysis. However, on direct immunofluorescence, in addition to the IgG deposition on the surface of the keratinocytes there is deposition of IgG and C3 complement at the dermoepidermal junction.

Antibodies in paraneoplastic pemphigus have been found to a variety of antigens. These include desmoplakins (constituents of the desmosomes), the bullous pemphigoid (BP) antigen 230 and, in some patients, to desmoglein 1 and desmoglein 3.

Clinically, PNP is linked to neoplasms, particularly lymphoproliferative disorders, but also thymomas, sarcomas and even carcinomas. Oral lesions are common and characteristically affect the vermillion border of the lips. The skin lesions often resemble erythema multiforme, with blisters and erosions on the upper trunk and erythematous target lesions on the palms and soles.

It is now generally accepted that PNP is not pemphigus, as the antibodies are directed against antigens other than desmogleins, and clinically it shows erythema multiforme-like lesions on the hands and feet. In addition, PNP is refractory to treatments that are usually effective in pemphigus. Removal of the neoplasms may induce a remission in some patients.

BENIGN FAMILIAL PEMPHIGUS (HAILEY–HAILEY DISEASE)

This disorder is sometimes referred to as benign familial pemphigus and is inherited as an autosomal dominant trait. It is not an autoimmune bullous disorder, but is characterized by epidermal splits and acantholytic cells. The disorder is due to a mutation of the ATPZC1 gene on chromosome 3q21. The gene is involved in changes in adhesion proteins and the assembly of adhesion junctions.

The lesions tend to appear in young adults, and sites of predilection are the neck, axillae (Figures 3.24 and 3.25) and groins. Characteristically, the lesions may begin as small blisters which rupture to form red crusted plaques. Lesions tend to spread peripherally to form larger plaques (Figure 3.24). One of the characteristic features is fissures within established plaques (Figure 3.25). Linear white bands may be present in the nails. The disease may run a protracted course but remissions can occur and the disease improves in old age.

Treatment

Because of the sites of involvement, secondary infection with bacteria and fungi is common. Specimens taken for bacteriology and mycology are helpful in the management.

Astringent lotions, such as magenta paint made up without the dye, can be effective, as the constituents are antibacterial and antifungal. Courses of systemic antibiotics may be necessary.

Topical corticosteroids are sometimes effective, but because of the moist sites are prone to lead to thinning of the skin and striae.

Loose-fitting clothing and avoidance of friction to the sites is important.

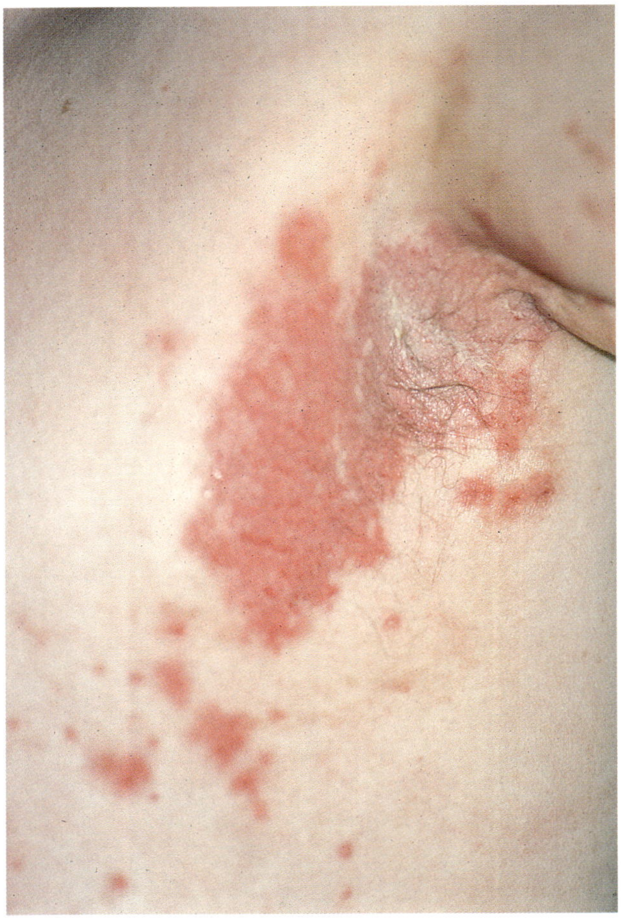

Figure 3.24 Large red moist plaque, formed by smaller lesions coalescing in the axilla, in benign familial pemphigus

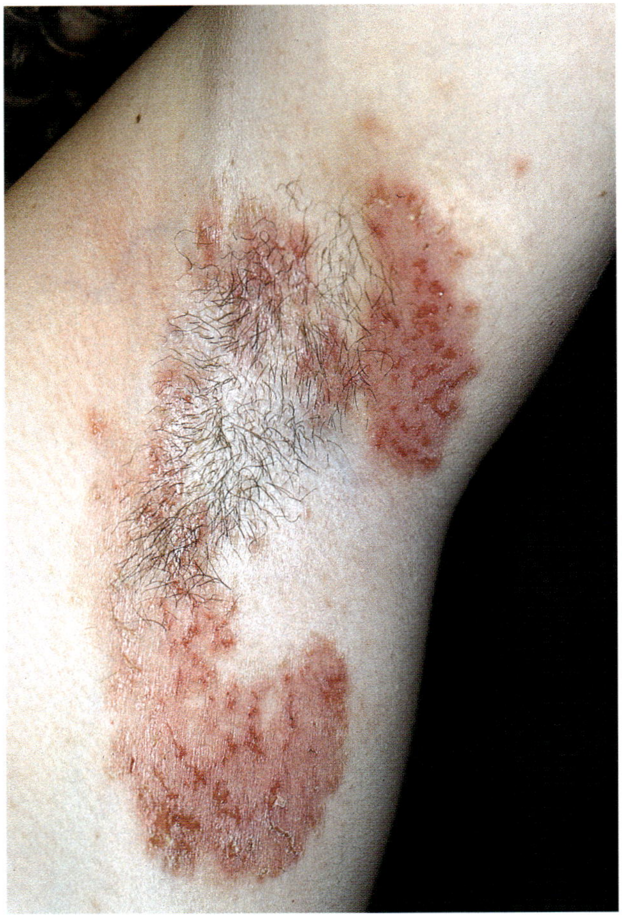

Figure 3.25 Characteristic fissures in a plaque in the axilla (benign familial pemphigus)

INTERCELLULAR IgA DERMATOSIS

The exact nosology of this entity has not been established. The characteristic feature is IgA on the surface of keratinocytes as distinct from IgG found in pemphigus. The antigen has not been determined, although desmoglein 1 and desmoglein 3 have been suggested. Circulating IgA antibodies to skin components have not been identified, and standard immunoblotting is negative.

Clinical features

IgA intercellular dermatosis has been reported in adults and children. Patients present with flaccid blisters or pustules arising on normal skin, or erythematous patches. The lesions may be pruritic and often have an annular configuration. The sites of predilection are the axillae and groins, although the face, trunk and proximal limbs may also be affected.

This dermatosis responds well to dapsone and sulfonamides but poorly to steroids. This suggests a possible role for neutrophils in the pathogenesis of the disease.

4 Dermoepidermal junction

The autoimmune subepidermal bullous disorders comprise a variety of recognized clinical entities, i.e. bullous pemphigoid, mucous membrane or cicatricial pemphigoid, linear immunoglobulin A (IgA) disease, acquired epidermolysis bullosa and pemphigoid gestationis. The autoantigens have now been identified for these disorders, although the reason why patients develop antibodies to these various antigens is unknown at present. Nevertheless, it has been suggested that autoimmune disease may be induced by infection[44].

Since the antigens are components of the basement membrane region, it is important to know its structure. On electron microscopy the basement membrane, which separates the epidermis and dermis, is composed of an upper translucent area, the lamina lucida, and an electron-dense region, the lamina densa (Figure 4.1). The basal layer of keratinocytes is attached to the basement membrane by electron-dense structures termed hemidesmosomes. The structures have an intracellular and an extracellular component. The latter consists of anchoring

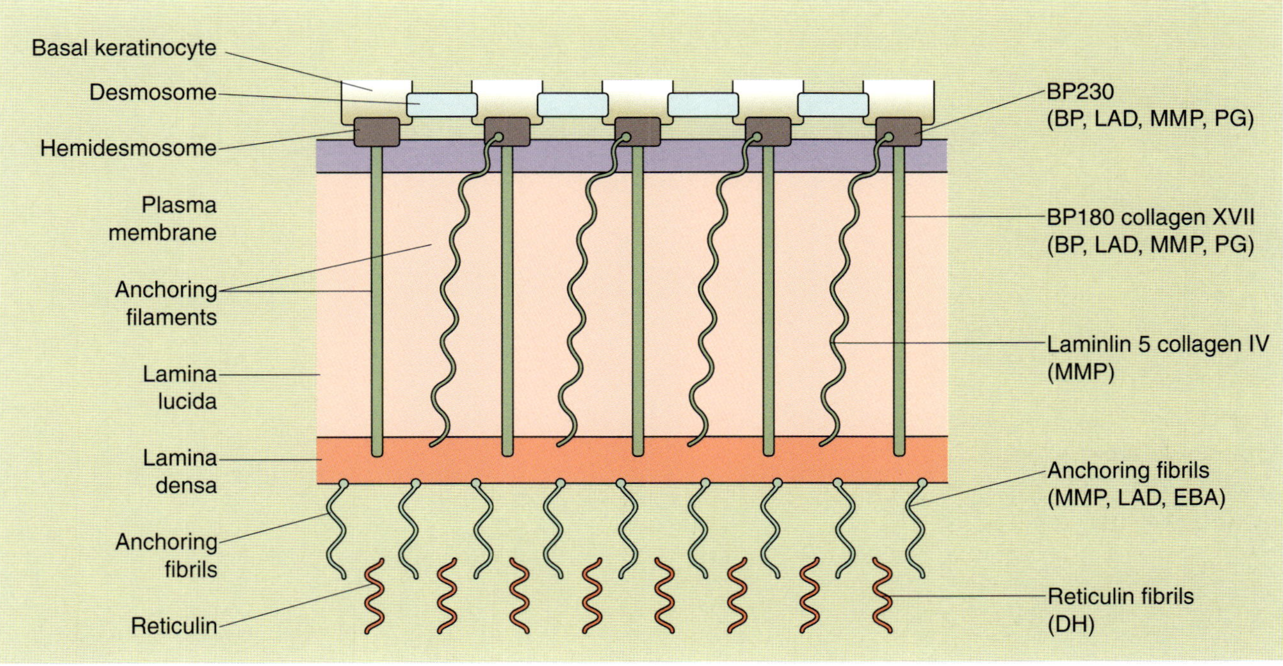

Figure 4.1 Antigenic sites in subepidermal bullous diseases. BP, bullous pemphigoid; LAD, linear IgA disease; MMP, mucous membrane pemphigoid; PG, pemphigoid gestationis; EBA, epidermolysis bullosa acquisita; DH, dermatitis herpetiformis

filaments which traverse the lamina lucida and end in the lamina densa, whose constituents include laminin 5 and type IV collagen. Below the lamina densa are anchoring fibrils composed of type VII collagen which anchor the lamina densa to the dermis.

The intracellular plaque of the hemidesmosome contains a polypeptide of 230 kDa known as bullous pemphigoid antigen 1 (BPAGl) or bullous pemphigoid 230 (BP230), one of the pemphigoid antigens, as a constituent of pemphigoid sera binds to it. The intracellular keratin filaments or tonofilaments are inserted into the hemidesmosomes, where they interact with BP230. The transmembrane components of the hemidesmosomes include BP180/collagen XVII or bullous pemphigoid antigen 2 (BPAG2) integrin. Bullous pemphigoid sera also bind to BP180, which has an intracellular component whereby the NH_2 terminal interacts with the same terminal of BP230, and also undergoes stabilizing interactions with plectins and β4 integrin. The long extracellular component of collagen XVII (BP180) is broken down by the action of proteases, and interacts with α6 integrin and with laminin 5 in the region of anchoring filaments. Laminin 5 also interacts with laminin isoforms and with integrins β4 and α6, as well as being the main ligand of type VII collagen, the major component of the anchoring fibrils in the dermis. Thus, there is a laminin bridge between the epidermal hemidesmosomes and the dermal matrix. Together these structures are known as the adhesion complex.

The antigens for the subepidermal bullous diseases that have been identified are components of the adhesion complex. When there is damage to these components, adherence between the epidermis and dermis is lost, and blister formation ultimately ensues. It has been shown that most of these antibodies can produce damage to the basement membrane region in the '*in vitro* situation'. The question that needs answering is: why are these antibodies produced before damage arises in the adherence complex, i.e. their production is the primary event, or are they produced secondary to damage in this region? Even if they are produced secondary to the damage they may still have the ability to be pathogenic and maintain the disease process.

5 Bullous pemphigoid

Bullous pemphigoid (BP) is one of the subepidermal immune-mediated bullous disorders. There is some overlap between these disorders, which will become apparent in the description of the clinical, pathological and pathogenetic mechanisms and treatment. These similarities and differences are discussed in Chapter 10.

INCIDENCE AND EPIDEMIOLOGY

Bullous pemphigoid is mainly a disease of the elderly, most commonly seen in persons over 60 years. However, it may occur in young persons including children. It is the most common immunobullous disorder in Western Europe. The incidence in France and Germany has been estimated as seven cases per million population per year[45,46]. A recent report from north-east Scotland has given the incidence at 14 per million per year[47]. A similar incidence was reported from Singapore[48]. In a survey of autoimmune bullous disorders over a 2-year period, the incidence of BP in 67 patients was 88%[48]. However, it has been claimed to be less common in other Chinese groups. In a study from Kuwait, the commonest autoimmune bullous disorder was pemphigus (47%), and the incidence of BP was 22%[49]. The incidence in other parts of the world is not known.

NATURAL HISTORY AND PROGNOSIS

BP has a considerably better outlook than does pemphigus. Before the advent of systemic steroids it was claimed that a spontaneous remission occurred on average after 2 years. The mortality rate of untreated pemphigoid is very low, but in treated disease with current drugs it is in the order of 10%, due to side-effects. Treatment suppresses the eruption but does not cure it, although spontaneous remission still occurs as in untreated patients.

ETIOLOGY

Genetic

There is no strong familial association in pemphigoid. In Europe, human leukocyte antigen (HLA)-DQ7 has been reported to be increased in men but not in women[50].

Other diseases

In the earlier literature it was said that BP may be associated with malignancy, particularly carcinoma of the stomach. However, more recent studies have not shown this association. It must be remembered that pemphigoid occurs in elderly patients who have an increased incidence of malignancy, the association being fortuitous. An incidence of malignancy in approximately 5% of BP patients has been reported from Italy, Japan and China, which is higher than in an age/sex-matched control group. However, screening for malignancy is not recommended.

Several other disorders have been reported to have a higher incidence in patients with BP, including psoriasis, diabetes mellitus, multiple sclerosis, rheumatoid arthritis and ulcerative colitis. What these diseases have in common is that they are thought to have an immunological basis.

Other triggers

Several drugs have been implicated in precipitating the disease, including penicillins, sulfonamides, penicillamine and frusemide. These drugs have been claimed to affect the immune system and allow induction of an autoimmune disease.

Trauma to the skin, with ultraviolet irradiation, thermal burns, radiotherapy and chemical irritants, has been associated with the triggering of BP. It is possible that damage to the skin releases antigens to which the body reacts with the production of autoantibodies.

PATHOLOGY

Histology

The blister in BP is subepidermal, with the roof of the blister being the epidermis (Figure 5.1). In the blister are neutrophils and eosinophils, and in the dermis there is an infiltrate of lymphocytes, histiocytes, neutrophils and eosinophils. Microabscesses are present in the dermal papillae adjacent to the blister, as seen in dermatitis herpetiformis.

Immunofluorescent studies

Direct immunofluorescent studies should be performed on perilesional skin, as the immunoglobulins may be destroyed by enzymes released from the cellular infiltrate. Immunoglobulin G (IgG) (Figure 5.2) and complement in lesional skin C3, or C3 alone, will be found along the line of the basement membrane. Split-skin techniques with 1 mol/l NaCl will allow separation of the epidermis from the dermis with the formation of a blister. The split occurs through the lamina lucida, and as the antigens in BP are associated with the hemidesmosomes, the IgG deposits are found in the roof of the blister (Figure 1.1).

Indirect immunofluorescence can be performed, and will reveal that about 75% of patients have circulating antibasement membrane antibodies. This investigation is not necessary routinely if direct immunofluorescence is positive.

PATHOGENESIS

The two major BP antigens are BP230 and BP180, and both are constituents of the hemidesmosomes. It is thought that binding of the antibody to BP180 is the first step in the development of a blister in BP[51].

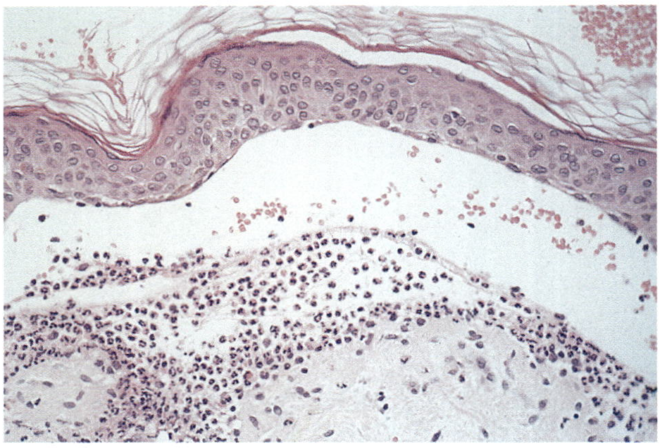

Figure 5.1 Subepidermal blister in bullous pemphigoid (BP) with infiltration of the blister by neutrophils and eosinophils

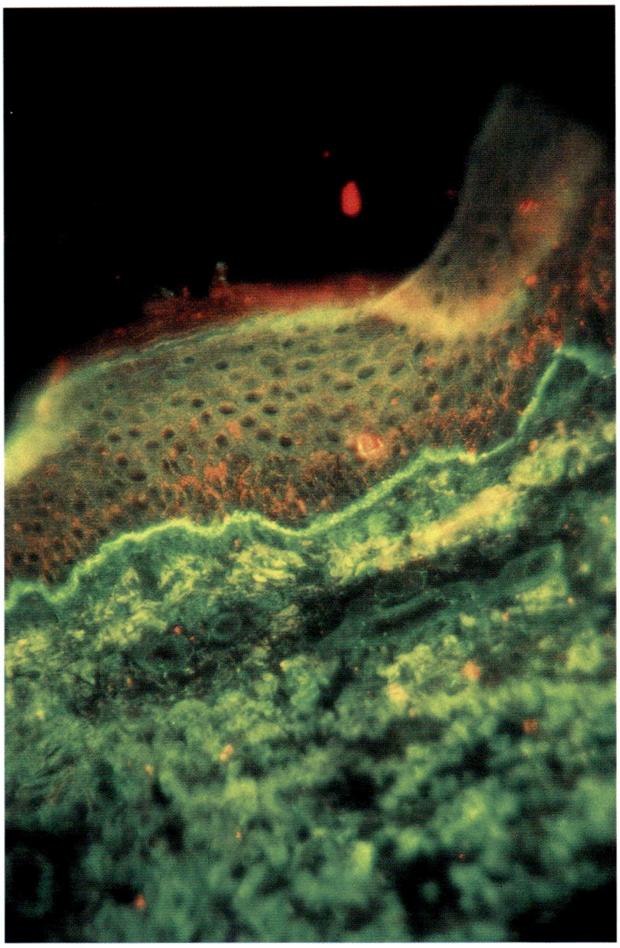

Figure 5.2 Immunoglobulin G (IgG) pemphigoid antibody (bright green) seen along the line of the basement membrane

BP230, also known as BPAG1, has a molecular weight of 230 kDa, is intracellular and is localized to the dense plaque (Figure 4.1). The portion of BP230 that is the target for the autoantibodies is located at the carboxy terminal, which mediates the interaction of keratin filaments and the hemidesmosome.

BP180, also known as collagen XVII (Figure 4.1), has a molecular weight of 180 kDa and is a transmembrane molecule with collagenous domains and an extracellular portion which is shed under physiological conditions. This extracellular component is the probable target for the antibodies.

The antibodies have been shown to be pathogenic in animal models, with the production of subepidermal blisters. It has also been shown in these animal models that complement is an essential part of the pathological process. Neutrophils play a crucial role in development of the blisters, as blister formation can be inhibited with an antineutrophil serum.

Thus the pathogenetic pathway is that antibodies bind to the BP antigens which activate complement. The complement components set off an inflammatory cascade attracting neutrophils, eosinophils and other inflammatory cells which release inflammatory mediators which, in turn, release lysomal enzymes and proteases cleaving the target antigens and damaging the hemidesmosomes. It is unknown why pathogenic antibodies are produced in an individual.

CLINICAL FEATURES

BP may commence in a number of ways. First, it may present as itchy urticarial plaques, usually on the limbs (Figures 5.3–5.5), and blisters appear on the urticarial plaques a few weeks later (Figures 5.3–5.5). Second, the initial lesions may present as itchy red scaly patches resembling eczema (Figure 5.6). In this presentation it may be some months before the blisters appear. Finally, BP can present as pruritus lasting up to 2–3 months before any skin lesions appear.

The blisters are tense and do not rupture easily as in pemphigus. The blisters vary in size from 0.5 to 2 cm. The urticarial plaques tend to be symmetrical (Figures 5.3 and 5.4). The commonest sites to be affected are the limbs (Figures 5.3–5.5), but the trunk may also be involved (Figures 5.6, 5.8 and 5.9). If the blisters rupture, erosions are formed (Figures 5.3–5.5 and 5.8). However, the blisters do not

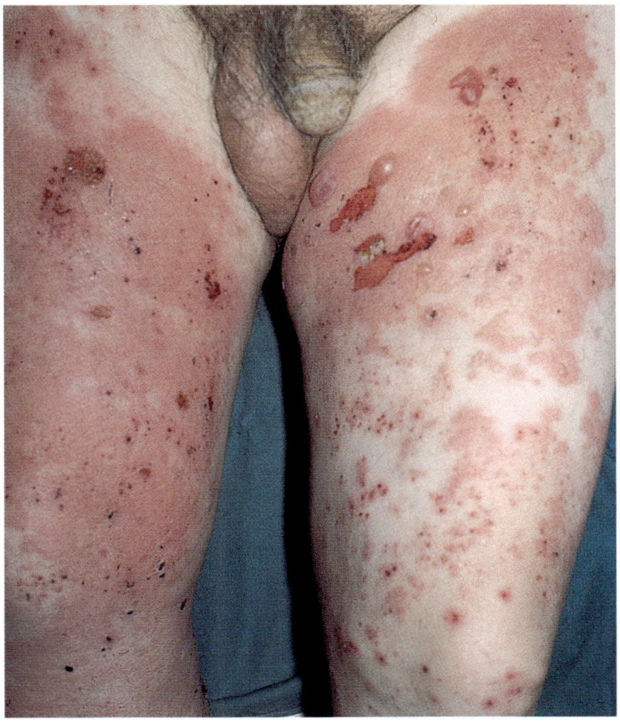

Figure 5.3 BP: symmetrical urticarial plaques on the thighs. Blisters and erosions from previous blisters are seen

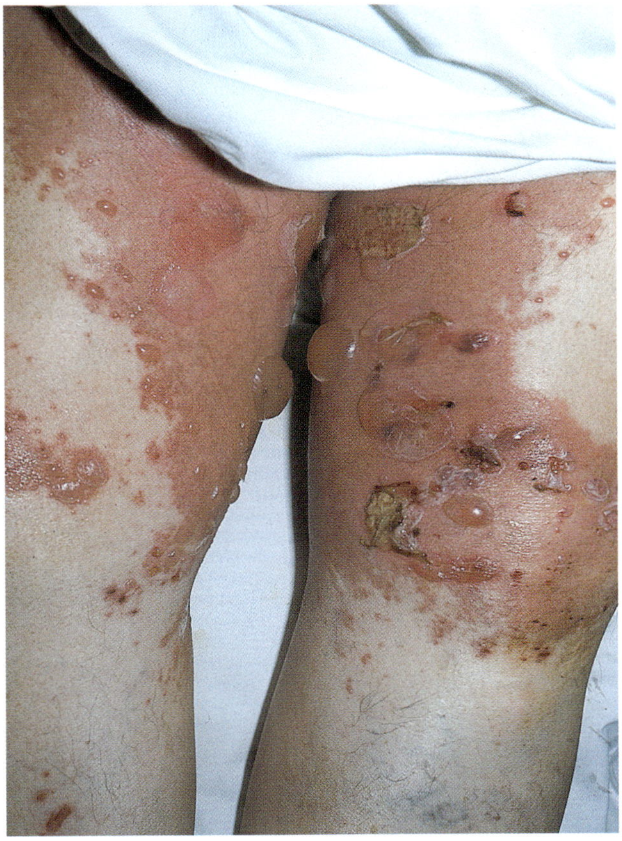

Figure 5.4 Symmetrical urticarial plaques with large tense blisters

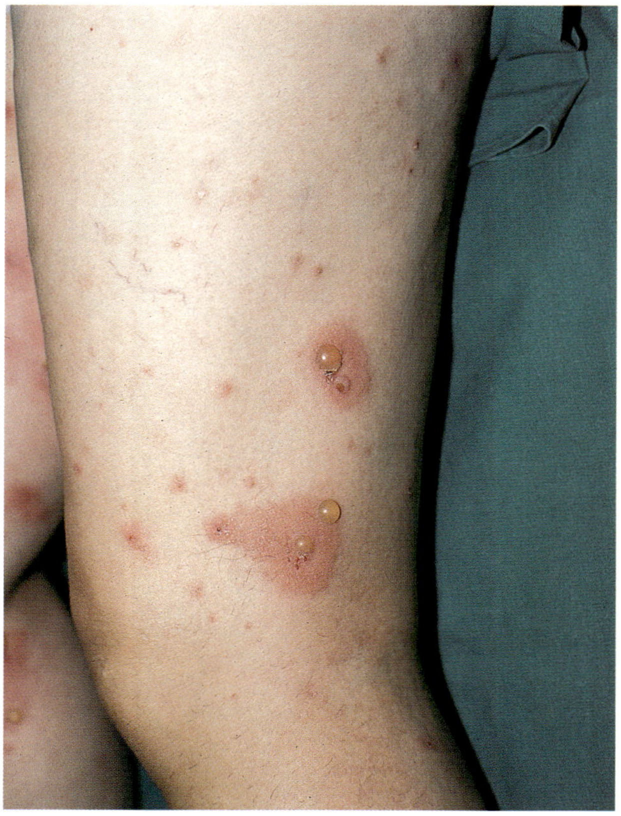

Figure 5.5 Small localized urticarial plaques with blisters in BP

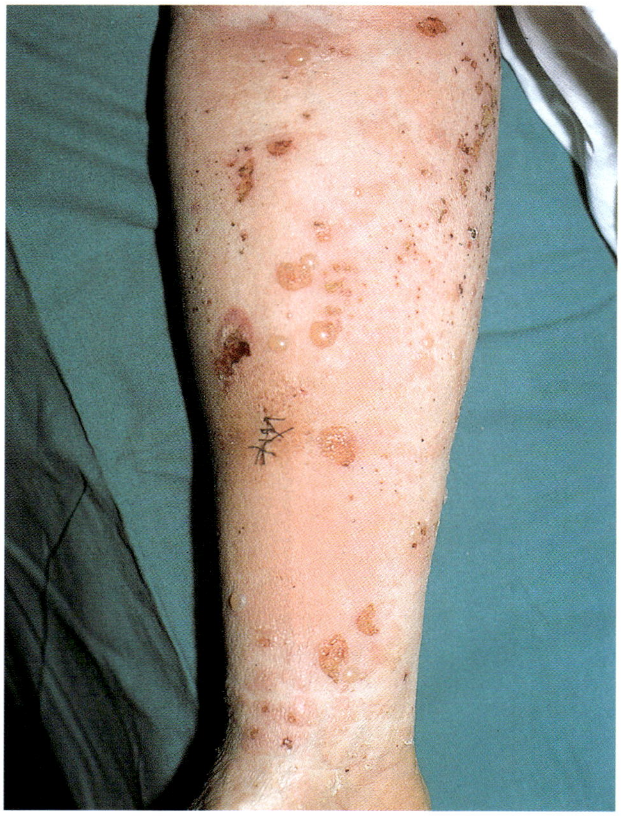

Figure 5.7 BP on the arm. Red areas with new blisters and some marks from previous blisters which have resolved

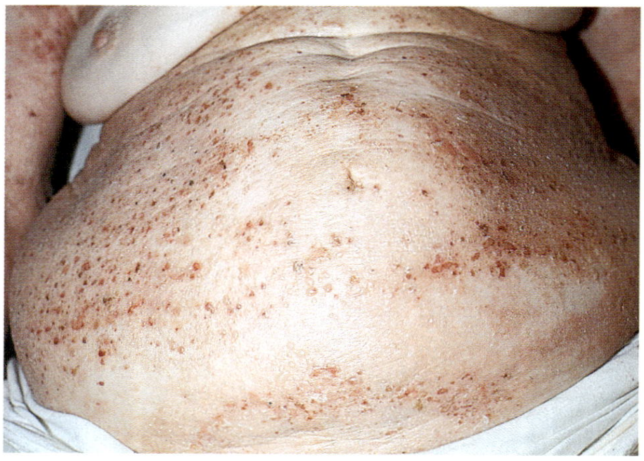

Figure 5.6 Red and scaly areas with excoriations on the abdomen. This presentation mimics eczema

always rupture, and the fluid is reabsorbed (Figures 5.10 and 5.11).

Apart from the blisters appearing on urticarial plaques or erythematous scaly areas, the blisters may arise on normal-looking skin (Figure 5.12). When the blisters resolve, the site may remain erythematous

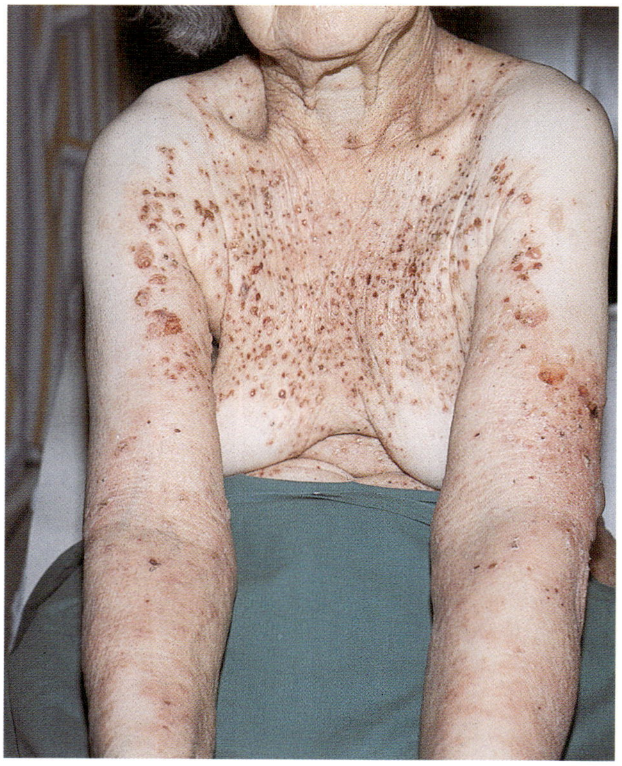

Figure 5.8 Extensive BP on the trunk and arms

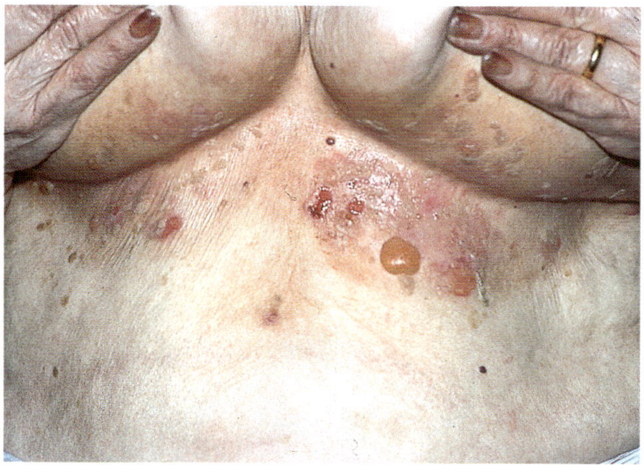

Figure 5.9 BP on the trunk localized in the infra-mammary area

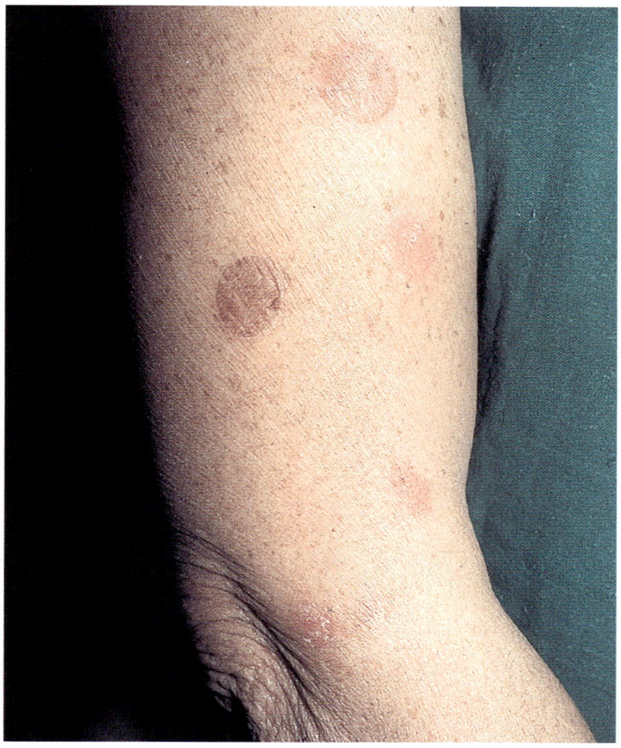

Figure 5.11 Resolving blisters. Some areas are red and others brown

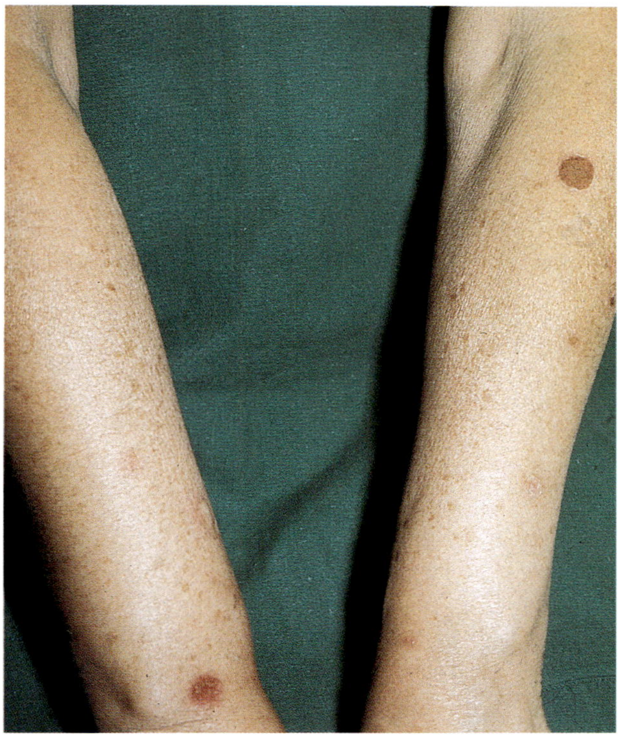

Figure 5.10 Resolving blisters on the arms in BP. Erythematous areas remain for a short time

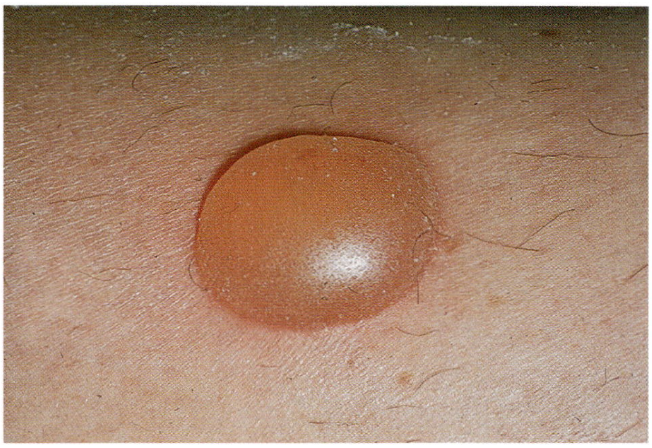

Figure 5.12 Large tense blisters in BP arising in normal-looking skin. No urticarial plaque present

for some weeks, and pigmentary changes, either hyper- or hypopigmentation (Figure 5.13), may occur particularly in dark-skinned individuals. However, scarring does not occur in BP. As with any blistering disease milia may form when the blisters resolve.

Localized pemphigoid is a clinical entity consisting of one or a group of lesions, usually on a lower leg (Figures 5.14 and 5.15). The condition may persist for months by itself, or other lesions may appear elsewhere on the trunk and limbs after many months.

Oral lesions have been reported but are less frequent than in pemphigus. The lesions are usually small blisters which rupture early due to the trauma of mastication. The question arises of how to distin-

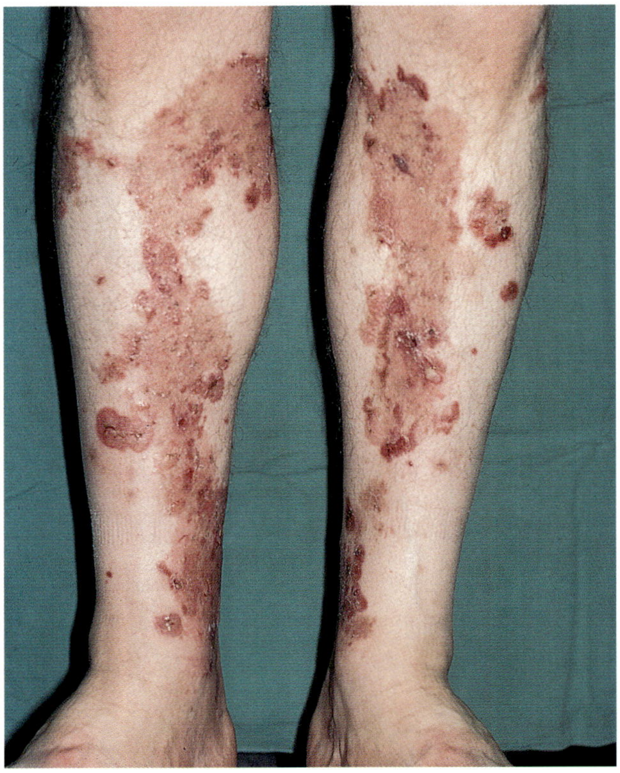

Figure 5.13 Resolving BP scabs are present at sites of previous erosions and there is post-inflammatory hyperpigmentation on the legs

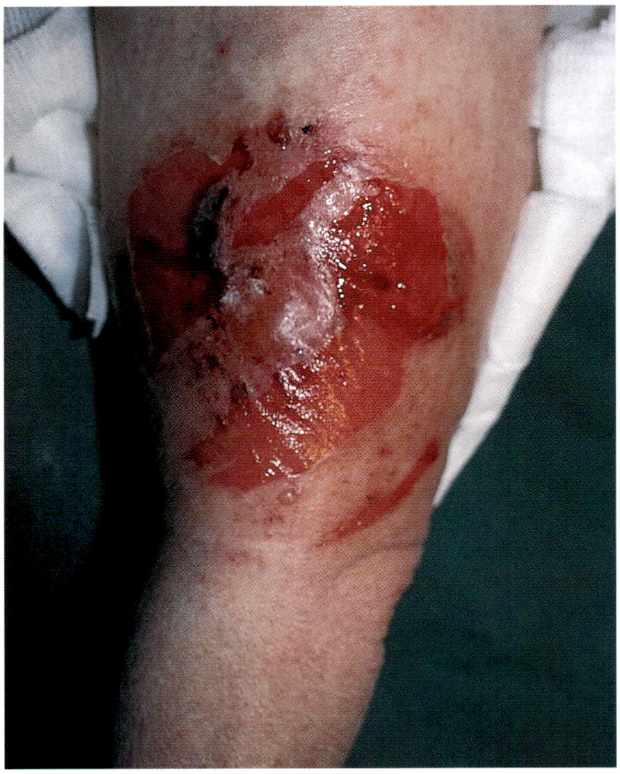

Figure 5.15 Large confluent erosion: localized pemphigoid

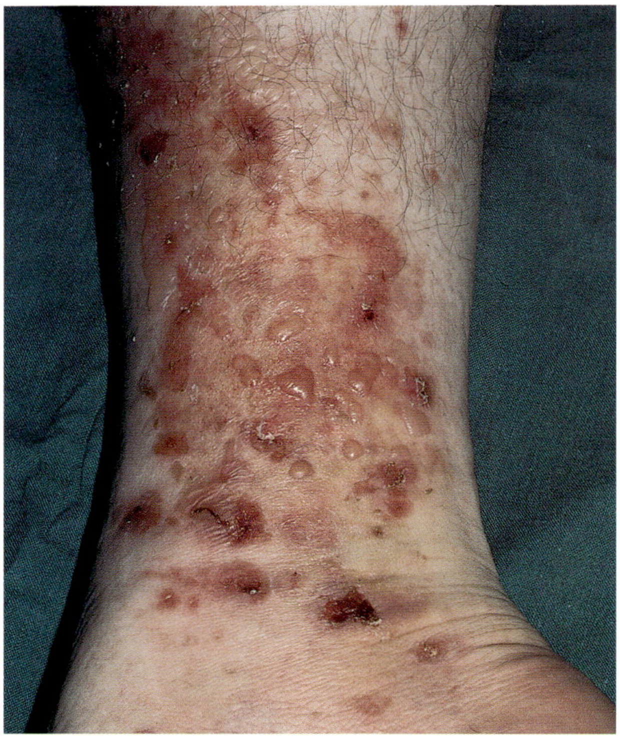

Figure 5.14 An area of localized pemphigoid above the ankle: blisters and scabbed erosions

guish pemphigoid with oral lesions from mucous membrane pemphigoid with skin lesions. It may simply have to be done based on which part is more severely affected. There seems to be some overlap between the two disorders, and hence both include pemphigoid in their name.

TREATMENT

Treatment is aimed at suppressing the lesions to an acceptable number.

Corticosteroids

These are the mainstay of treatment and may be used topically or systemically. Only very potent (group IV) topical steroids are likely to have any clinical effect, and should be used for localized pemphigoid or when very few lesions are present in generalized disease.

Systemic corticosteroids are usually effective in relatively small doses, compared with pemphigus. If the patient is very elderly then an initial dose of prednisolone 20 mg daily should be given. If patients are younger, 60–80 years, and their general health is good then an initial dose of 30–40 mg daily is appropriate. It should be stressed that BP *per se* has a relatively good prognosis and a very low mortality rate. However, the current mortality rate with treatment is approximately 10%, and most cases of death are treatment-related.

Once control of the disease has been achieved, the dose of prednisolone should be gradually reduced, i.e. by 5–10 mg daily per month. If lesions start to reappear then no further reduction of dose should be attempted and other treatment modalities considered if the dose has not been reduced to 15 mg daily or less. It should be remembered that the average duration of BP before remission occurs is 2 years, so if maintenance of the steroid is relatively low, i.e. below 15 mg daily, then other drugs may not be required. The decision should be based on the individual's general health, other disorders and the side-effects of systemic steroids that have occurred or are likely to occur.

OTHER DRUGS

Other drugs used for BP are immunosuppressive and include azathioprine, mycophenolate mofetil, methotrexate and cyclosporine. These are used as steroid-sparing drugs. (The dose and side-effects are given in the 'Treatment' section of Chapter 3.) Most experience has been with azathioprine. It should be stressed that it takes 6–8 weeks before any clinical effect is seen. Once no new lesions appear the dose of steroid can be gradually decreased by 1 mg/day every 2 weeks to 5 mg daily. If the patient remains clear, then the dose of immunosuppressive drugs can also be gradually reduced. The dose of drugs is then titrated up or down according to the clinical state, and, if possible, the dose of systemic steroid should be maintained below 7.5 mg daily of prednisolone.

PROGNOSIS AND NATURAL HISTORY

BP has a good prognosis, the average duration before remission occurs being 2 years. Treatments used to control the disease are associated with relatively high morbidity, and it has been estimated that the mortality rate of 10% is related to treatment and not the disease *per se*.

DIFFERENTIAL DIAGNOSIS

In the early phase of BP when no blisters are present, it may be difficult to make the diagnosis. Patients with only pruritus have to be distinguished from those with other causes of pruritus without a significant rash, e.g. liver disease, lymphoma, low-grade eczema and psychogenic disorders. When only urticarial plaques are present then it has to be distinguished from urticaria. In the latter, the lesions last for only a few hours before they disappear and are replaced by new lesions, whereas the urticarial plaques in BP persist for days or weeks. When red scaly lesions are the presenting features, then BP must be distinguished from eczema, psoriasis and cutaneous T-cell lymphoma. If the presenting feature is urticarial or red and scaly, a biopsy from perilesional skin for direct immunofluorescence is the best method of establishing the diagnosis. If only pruritus is present, unless BP is included in the differential diagnosis it is unlikely that the diagnosis will be made until lesions appear.

In the bullous phase, then BP has to be distinguished from the other immunobullous disorders. The fact that BP usually presents in the elderly is an important feature, as most of the others present earlier. Dermatitis herpetiformis usually begins in younger persons, and has characteristic sites of involvement, i.e. extensor surface of the elbows and forearms, buttocks and extensor surface of the knees. In pemphigus the blisters are flaccid and rupture easily, and the patient may present with erosions rather than blisters. Linear IgA disease usually starts at an earlier age. The blisters tend to be smaller and often affect the intertriginous regions. The blisters may also be found at the edges of a crusted lesion, sometimes referred to as a 'crown of jewels'. Mucous membrane lesions are commoner in linear IgA disease than in BP. The disorder which may be the most difficult to distinguish on clinical grounds is mucous membrane pemphigoid if the skin is involved extensively. The most reliable way to establish the correct diagnosis is by direct immunofluorescence. However, even then difficulties may arise, as IgA deposition in BP has been described and both IgG and IgA may be found in mucous membrane pemphigoid. IgG is not usually found in linear IgA disease, and thus the distinction between this disorder and BP is easier to make.

6 Linear IgA disease

Linear IgA disease (LAD) was recognized as a definitive entity in the late 1970s. Previously it was grouped as a variant of dermatitis herpetiformis (DH), as immunoglobulin A (IgA) was present in uninvolved skin and the eruption responded to dapsone. However, it was noted that patients with the homogeneous linear pattern of IgA deposition along the line of the basement membrane (Figure 6.1) had clinical features which distinguished them from DH, the most important of which were a different distribution of the eruption and the fact that patients with LAD did not have an associated gluten-sensitive enteropathy. Clinically there are two distinct entities of LAD: the adult and the childhood disorders. Whether they are actually two separate entities with regard to etiology and pathogenesis is yet to be determined. The clinical features are described below separately, but the others together.

INCIDENCE AND EPIDEMIOLOGY

LAD is a relatively rare bullous disease with an incidence of 0.5–1.3 per million per year in European countries[45,46], and the adult variety is more common than the childhood one. It has been reported to be more common in Asian countries, although recent studies from Singapore[48] reported an incidence of 0.26 and from Kuwait of 0.69 per million per year[49]. However, LAD is more common in mainland China where one-third of all subepidermal bullous diseases is LAD, and one-third of these occurs in children[52]. There is also a higher proportion of childhood LAD in other parts of South-East Asia and in Blacks in South Africa than in European countries.

ETIOLOGY

Genetic

There is an association between LAD and the extended haplotype human leukocyte antigen HLA-B8/CW7/DR3, which is also associated with early onset.

Environmental factors

The factor most strongly associated is prior antibiotic use. This has been reported in 25% of patients[53]. The antibiotics most commonly incriminated are penicillins and vancomycin.

However, it is possible that the infection for which the antibiotics were taken initiated the disease.

PATHOLOGY

Histology

This is similar to that of pemphigoid and dermatitis herpetiformis. A subepidermal blister is the predominant feature, which contains neutrophils and eosinophils. Dermal papillary microabscesses are also present. A lymphocyte/histiocyte infiltrate is present in the dermis.

Immunofluorescent studies

Direct immunofluorescence is the most reliable test for establishing the diagnosis. As with other bullous disorders, the biopsy should be taken from uninvolved perilesional skin as the immunoglobulin deposits are destroyed within the blister region.

Immunofluorescence shows a linear homogeneous band of IgA along the basement region (Figure 6.1). IgG, IgM and C3 complement have also been found at the same site and in the same pattern. The split-skin test shows that, although in the majority of patients the IgA deposits are in the roof, in a few the deposits are in the floor of the blister, i.e. the lamina densa or dermal components. IgA deposits are also found in the oral mucosa and sometimes in the conjunctiva[54]. Immunoelectron microscopy has confirmed that the IgA deposits are in the hemidesmosome region or in the lamina densa. However, the clinical features do not show a difference with the different sites of IgA deposition.

Indirect immunofluorescence reveals circulating antibodies in only 30% of adults but in 80% of children. As with direct immunofluorescence, the antibodies bind to the hemidesmosome region in the majority of patients, but in some the binding is to the lamina densa region.

PATHOGENESIS

The antibodies in LAD are IgA, usually IgA1, and monomeric. In DH, however, the IgA deposits are dimeric, arising from the intestine, and this difference could be used to distinguish the two diseases if the IgA deposits are linear in DH, although the linear IgA deposits in DH are not homogeneous.

The IgA antibodies are mainly directed to the BP180 antigen, although antibodies to BP230 may also be present as well as to a unique antigen LAD285 (with a molecular weight of 285 kDa). The dermal antigens could be the shed domain of the anchoring filaments which reach to the lamina densa. These antigens have molecular weights of 97 and 120 kDa. In addition there are antibodies to anchoring fibrils (collagen VII) which are localized to the lamina densa and upper dermis.

Why these antibodies form is not known, nor is the primary initiating factor in LAD. There is some evidence that the antibodies found in LAD are pathogenic in that they cause skin splitting in culture.

CLINICAL FEATURES

Adult disease

Both the skin and the mucous membranes may be affected. The disorder may occur at any age after puberty, and it is not uncommon in the elderly.

LAD may begin with pruritus before any skin lesions appear, similar to pemphigoid, or it may present with skin lesions. The lesions have no specific site of predilection and may occur on the trunk (Figures 6.2 and 6.3), limbs (Figures 6.4 and 6.5), face

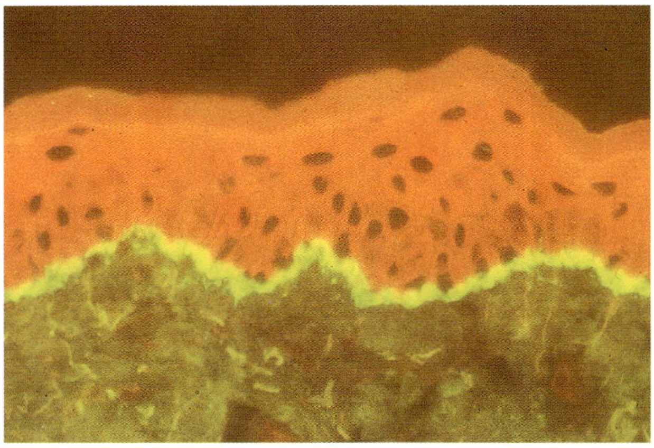

Figure 6.1 Linear homogeneous band of immunoglobulin A (IgA) along the line of the basement membrane

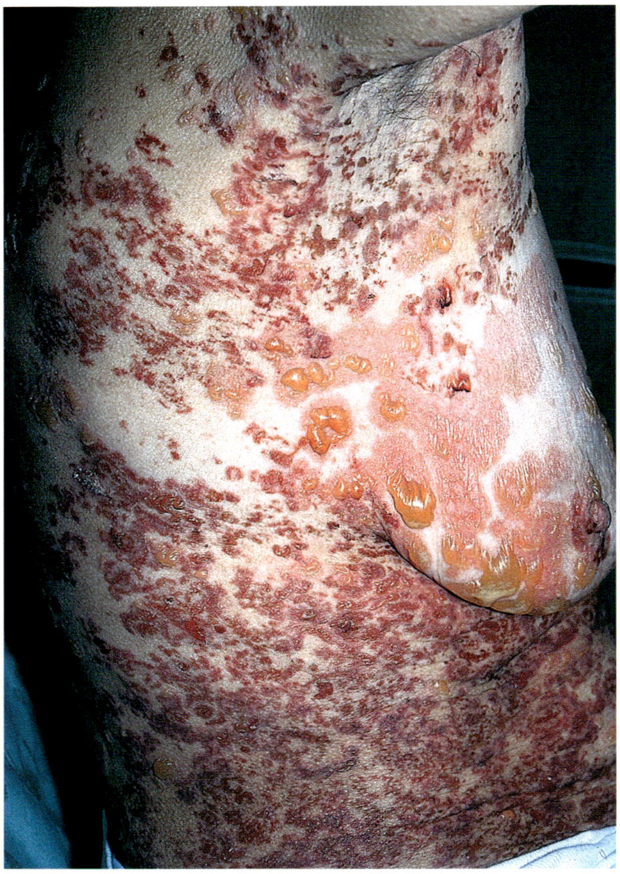

Figure 6.2 Extensive involvement of the trunk in linear IgA disease (LAD)

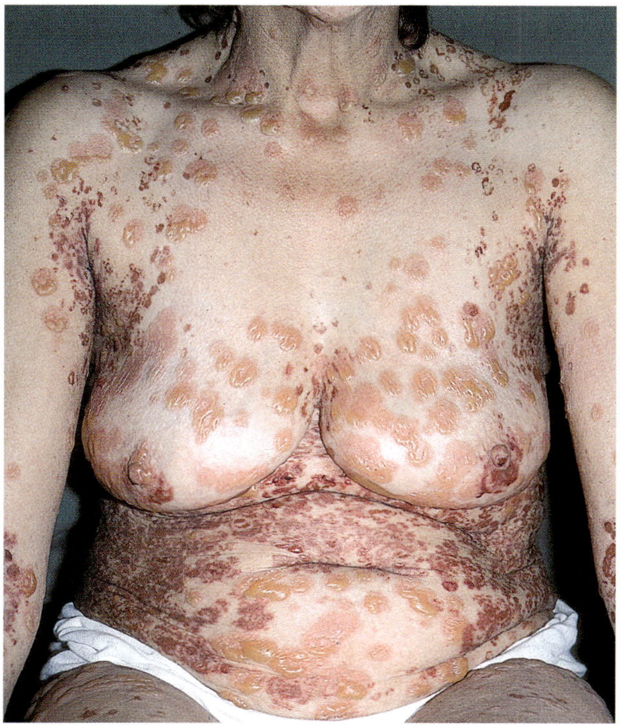

Figure 6.3 Involvement of the trunk

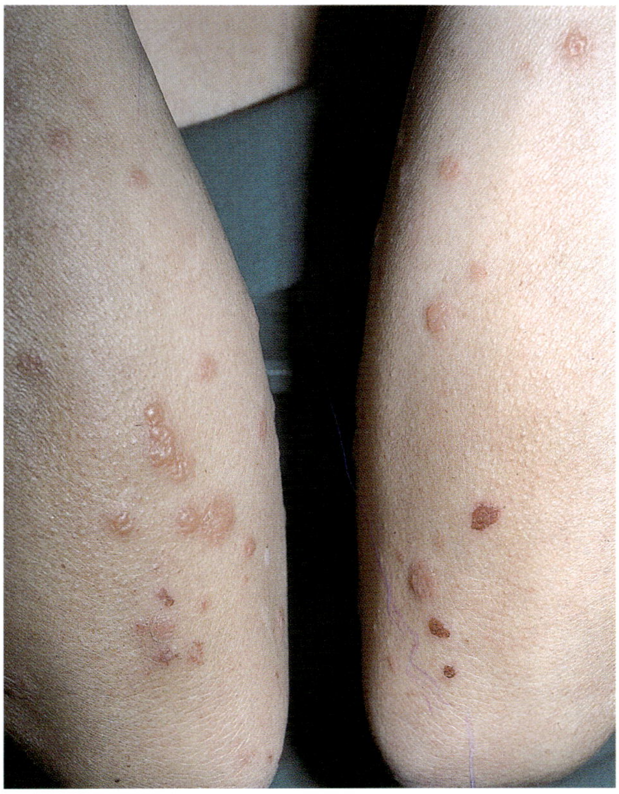

Figure 6.4 LAD on extensor surface of the arms. This must be distinguished from dermatitis herpetiformis which characteristically involves the point of the elbows and usually only the proximal third of the forearm

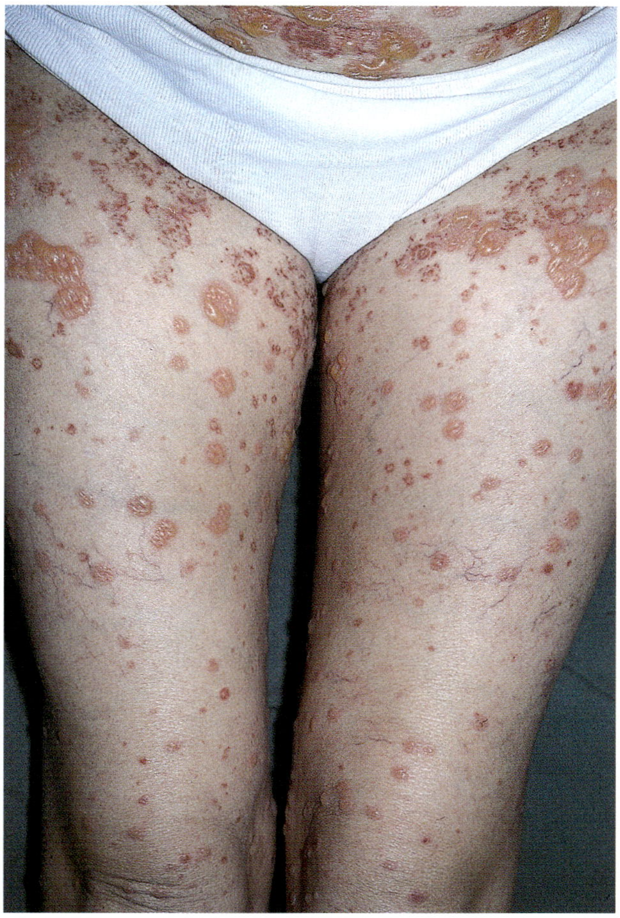

Figure 6.5 Lesions on thighs

and scalp (Figure 6.6). Involvement of intertriginous areas, particularly the groins (Figure 6.7) and axillae (Figure 6.8), is common. As with other skin disorders which have an 'endogenous' pathogenetic basis, the eruption is symmetrical (Figures 6.4 and 6.5). Urticarial plaques are common and the blisters arise from these (Figures 6.2–6.5), or they may occur from normal-looking skin. The blisters may be solitary or arranged in an annular fashion around the edges of a red urticarial plaque (Figures 6.3, 6.5 and 6.9), which is a fairly characteristic feature, and this type of lesion has been referred to as a 'crown of jewels'. Crusts and scabs are common. Often, the center of the annulus becomes crusted and scabbed (Figure 6.10). Large erosions that occur in pemphigus and sometimes in bullous pemphigoid are not usually seen. The blisters are relatively small (0.5–1.0 cm) compared with those that may be seen in pemphigoid.

Involvement of the mucous membranes is not uncommon. In the mouth there will be erosions and ulcers, and they may involve the buccal mucosae,

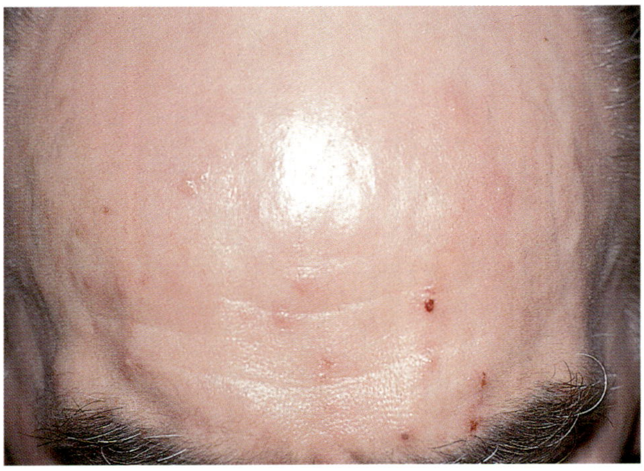

Figure 6.6 Small blisters and papules, some excoriations on the forehead and scalp

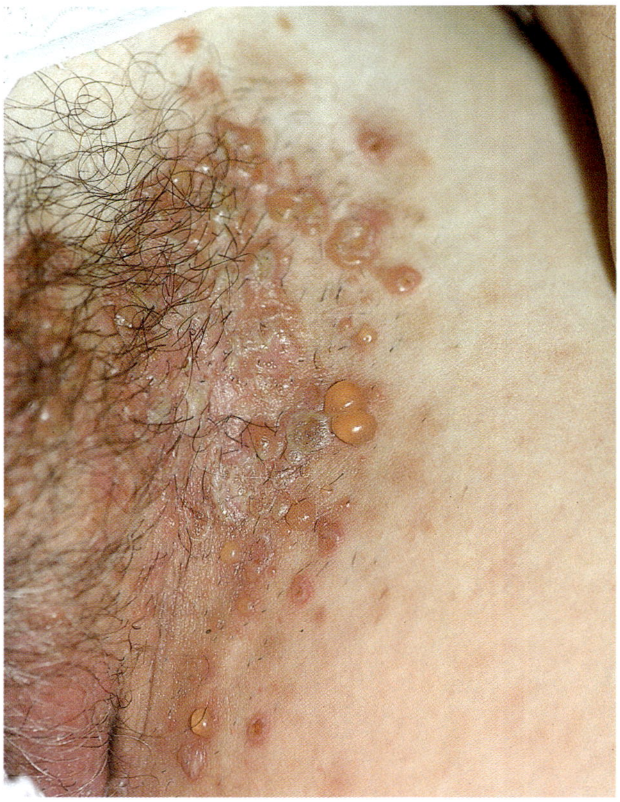

Figure 6.7 Lesions in groin

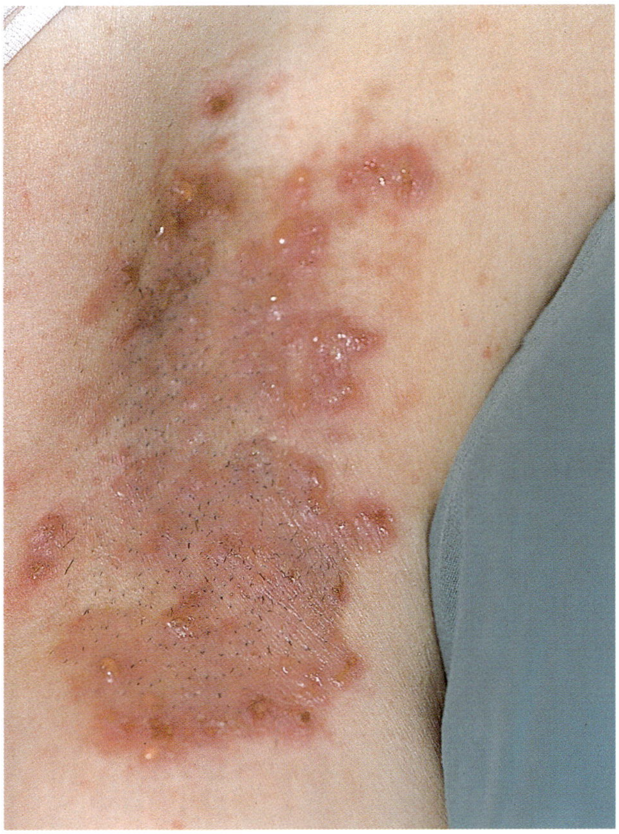

Figure 6.8 Involvement of axilla

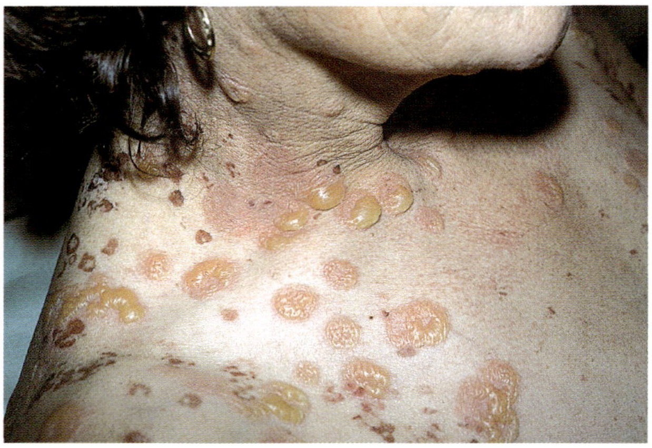

Figure 6.9 Blisters occurring at the periphery of urticarial plaques, giving an annular configuration

tongue (Figure 6.11), lips (Figure 6.12) and palate. The pharynx, larynx and esophagus may be involved, presenting as hoarseness and dysphagia, respectively. The nasal mucosa, if affected, presents with crusting, congestion and bloody discharge. The conjunctiva can be affected and the features are similar to those of mucous membrane pemphigoid (MMP). The involvement may begin as soreness and/or redness. This may progress to scarring (Figure 6.13), and if progressive to blindness. The genitalia can be involved with ulcers, erosions and eventual scarring (Figure 6.14).

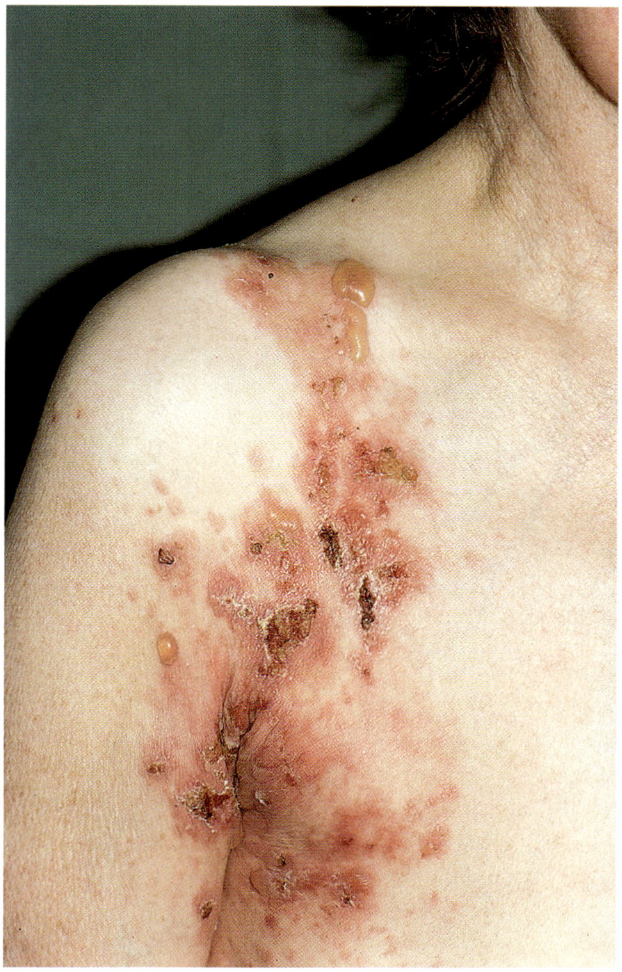

Figure 6.10 Crusts and scabs in resolving lesions. Some blisters still present at the periphery

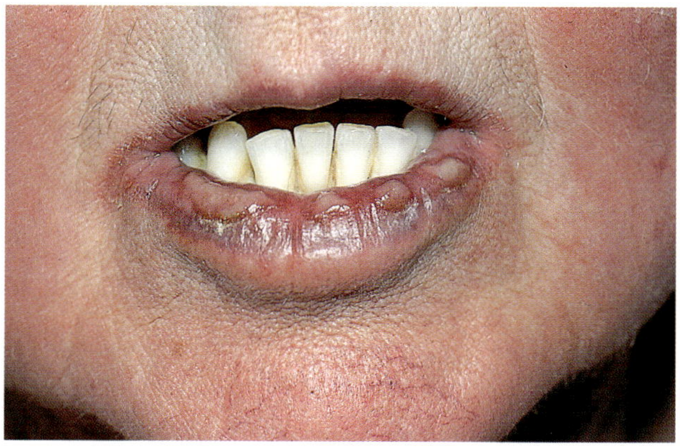

Figure 6.12 Ulcers on the labial mucosal surface

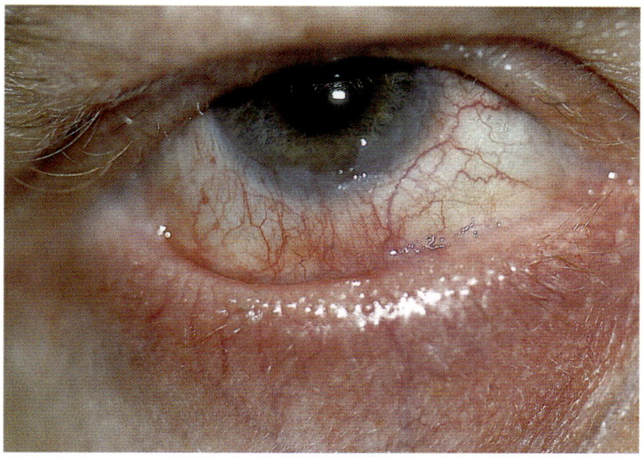

Figure 6.13 Scarring of the conjunctiva in LAD

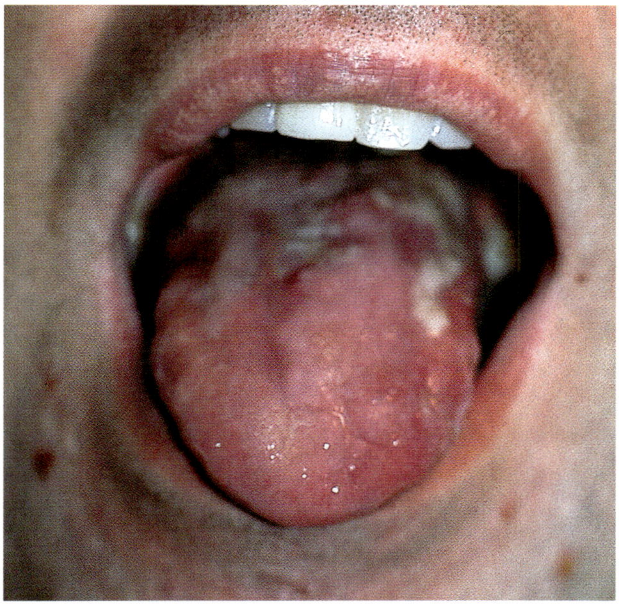

Figure 6.11 Erosions on the tongue in LAD

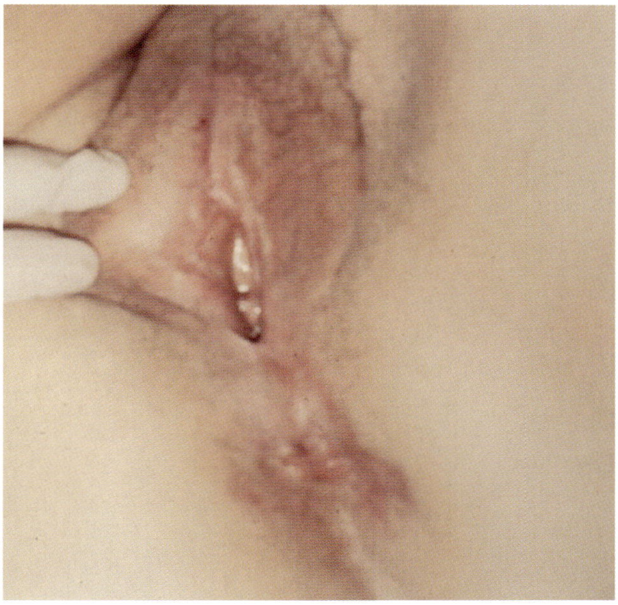

Figure 6.14 Scarring of the vulva due to LAD (with kind permission of Professor F. Wojnarowska)

Childhood disease

This was previously termed chronic bullous disease of childhood. Males and females seem to be similarly affected. Childhood LAD usually begins before the age of 5 and may commence before the age of 2 years. The commonest sites of involvement are the pubic area and around and on the genitalia (Figures 6.15 and 6.16) and the perioral region of the face. The eruption may spread to involve the trunk and limbs. The lesions usually commence as urticarial papules and plaques, and the blisters often appear at the edges of the plaques in an annular configuration. Occasionally the blisters arise from normal-looking skin.

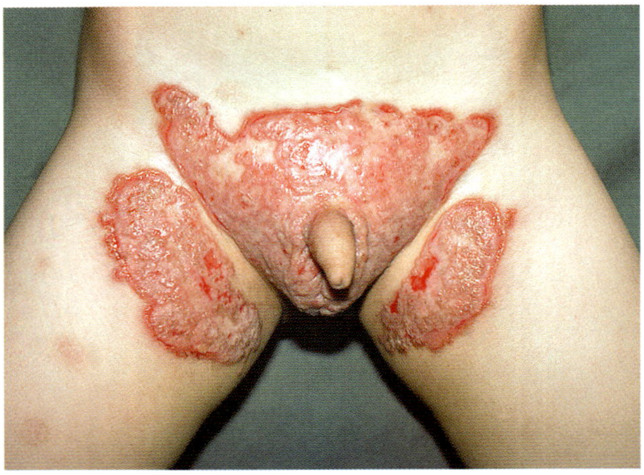

Figure 6.15 LAD in childhood. The commonest site is the pubic area and genitalia

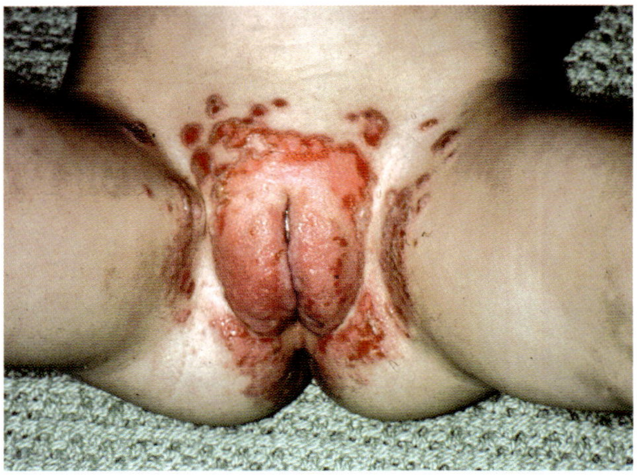

Figure 6.16 Blisters and scabs on the genitalia, groins and thighs in childhood LAD (with kind permission of Professor F. Wojnarowska)

Mucosal involvement is common, but does not always occur. In the mouth there may be painful ulcers and erosions. Involvement of the eyes presents with redness and soreness and, as in adults, may progress to scarring.

Nasal involvement presents with congestion and discharge which may be bloody.

Pharyngeal and laryngeal lesions may give rise to dysphagia and hoarseness, respectively.

TREATMENT

As the prognosis is good in the majority of individuals, over-treatment with systemic drugs should be avoided.

Dapsone

LAD, both adult and childhood, responds well to dapsone, which is why LAD was considered to be DH before immunofluorescent studies made the distinction possible between the two diseases.

Prior to using dapsone, patients who may be at risk of glucose-6-phosphate dehydrogenase (G-6-PD) deficiency should be tested for this possibility. G-6-PD deficiency is genetically determined, and is most commonly seen in persons from the Middle East. It will lead to severe hemolysis if dapsone is taken.

The initial dose of dapsone in adults is 50 mg daily. After a week, the dose may be titrated up or down depending on the clinical response and side-effects. The increase or decrease should be stepwise. The maximum dose should not exceed 300 mg/day. As the 50-mg tablet is the lowest strength available, the dose can be decreased by lengthening the number of days between taking the tablets. In children the initial starting dose is 0.5 mg/kg/day, and the dapsone tablets may have to be broken in two to obtain a small dose and given on alternate days.

Apart from hemolysis, the side-effects of dapsone include methemoglobinemia, peripheral neuropathy, headache, depression, agranulocytosis and, rarely, the dapsone syndrome (lymphadenopathy and hepatitis).

Thus, patients taking dapsone should be monitored after the first week and then every 2 weeks for the next month and then monthly for 3 months. Hematological side-effects are usually seen in the first 3 months. However, patients on long-term treatment should be seen at least twice a year.

Sulfonamides

If patients are unable to take dapsone then either sulfapyridine or sulfamethoxypyridazine may be given. The initial dose of the former for an adult is 2 g per day, and 1 g per day for the latter. The dose may then be titrated up or down to achieve control of the eruption on the smallest possible dose. The maximum dose for sulfapyridine is 4 g per day, and is 1.5 g per day for sulfamethoxypyridazine. Side-effects of sulfonamides include drug eruptions and agranulocytosis.

In the elderly it is advisable to initiate treatment with a sulfonamide, as the incidence of side-effects is less than with dapsone. Although young adults tolerate a small degree of hemolysis, elderly subjects may not.

If side-effects occur with a high dose of dapsone or sulfonamides required to control the eruption, then combining dapsone with a sulfonamide or a sulfonamide with another sulfonamide may allow control of the rash without side-effects.

Other drugs

Systemic corticosteroids

These are sometimes required to control the mucous membrane lesions in addition to dapsone and/or sulfonamides. A relatively low dose, i.e. 5–10 mg daily, should be aimed for.

Antibiotics

Good results have been obtained with erythromycin in children[55]. Tetracyclines have also been claimed to be helpful, but are often combined with nicotinamide to improve results.

Colchicine has been used in both children and adults with favorable results.

It should be stressed that the majority of patients, both children and adults, have a good prognosis, and thus if good control of the eruption has been achieved then a gradual reduction in drug requirements should be attempted at follow-up visits.

PROGNOSIS AND NATURAL HISTORY

LAD has a relatively good prognosis in both the childhood and adult forms.

Most children have a permanent remission before puberty. However, there are now reports of the disease extending into adult life[56]. In adult LAD the majority have a remission within 3–6 years. There is a suggestion that patients with severe mucous membrane involvement have more persistent disease. It is possible that these patients have linear IgA mucous membrane pemphigoid rather than LAD.

ASSOCIATED DISEASES

An increase in ulcerative colitis[57] and lymphoproliferative disorders[58] in adults has been reported. The latter have been reported in patients whose LAD eruption has gone into remission.

DIFFERENTIAL DIAGNOSIS

LAD has to be distinguished from other bullous diseases. As the bullae are subepidermal, they are tense and do not rupture as easily as pemphigus blisters. If LAD presents late in life then it has to be distinguished from bullous pemphigoid (BP). If there is severe involvement of the mucous membranes then a distinction has to be made from mucous membrane pemphigoid (MMP). The distinction of LAD from other autoimmune bullous diseases may be made by direct immunofluorescent studies. The distinction between LAD and IgA mucous membrane pemphigoid may be the most difficult. In this instance, it has been proposed that that the disease should be classified as mucous membrane pemphigoid. Conversely, there are so-called 'mixed' immunobullous disorders (see Chapter 10), with both linear IgG and IgA deposits along the basement membrane region. In these cases the course of the disease is usually more like LAD, and has a good response to dapsone and sulfonamides. The exact nosology of this group of patients is unclear, but the natural history is that of LAD.

The 'non-bullous' disorders that may pose diagnostic problems are bullous impetigo and papular urticaria. In the former, the blisters rupture more easily and crusted lesions and erosions are usually present. Bacteriology should easily distinguish impetigo from LAD.

Severe reactions to insect bites may present with tense blisters which are widespread. If the source of the insects is not identified and dealt with, the disease may become chronic. Immunofluorescent studies are the most appropriate way to determine the correct diagnosis.

7 Pemphigoid gestationis

Pemphigoid gestationis (PG) was originally referred to as herpes gestationis, but as the immunofluorescent findings were similar to those of bullous pemphigoid the name was changed.

EPIDEMIOLOGY

PG is a rare disease. In Caucasians it has been reported to occur in 1 : 10 000[59] and 1 : 60 000 pregnancies[60]. The incidence in Western Europe has been estimated at 0.5 per million per year. It has been reported in Blacks, and the human leukocyte antigen (HLA) haplotype in one Black was that found in Caucasians with PG, i.e. B8/DR3/DR4. It is rare in the Far East, and no case was found in Singapore over a 2-year period in which 67 patients presented with subepidermal bullous disease[48]. However, in a study of bullous disorders from Kuwait, it was found to be the third commonest bullous disease, accounting for 19% of all bullous disorders; pemphigus was the most common at 42%, followed by pemphigoid at 22%[49].

ETIOLOGY

PG is dependent on paternally derived antigens which are present in the fetus, and occasionally in a hydatidiform mole or choriocarcinoma. There is a higher incidence of HLA-DR2 in fathers compared with the general population. It is thought that, because of differences in HLA antigens between mother and fetus, an immune response is triggered which results in damage to the maternal skin. There is evidence of immune activation in the placenta and of placental insufficiency.

Mothers have a high incidence of the HLA haplotype B8/DR3/DR4, which is associated with autoimmune disorders. They also have a high incidence of the C4-null allele, which is in linkage disequilibrium with the B8/DR3/DR4 haplotype. This association is related to poor clearance of immune complexes, which may be relevant to the development of PG.

PATHOLOGY

The bullous lesions are subepidermal. Preceding blister formation there is edema of the dermal papillae and infiltration with eosinophils, forming a papillary microabscess. Eosinophils also infiltrate into the epidermis, and spongiosis is also present. In addition there is a perivascular infiltrate of lymphocytes and histiocytes common to subepidermal bullous dermatoses.

Direct immunofluorescent studies show C3 complement bound to the basement membrane region in all patients, and immunoglobulin G (IgG) may also be found at the same site. With more refined immunofluorescent techniques, IgG can be found in all biopsies. Both C3 and IgG have also been found in the placenta and uninvolved skin. Indirect immunofluorescent studies show that serum contains a factor which binds C3 to the basement membrane (Figure 7.1). This factor was termed the HG factor when the disorder was known as 'herpes' gestationis.

The split-skin technique has shown the IgG to be bound to the roof of the blister, i.e. the epidermal side. Immunoelectron microscopy has shown deposits in the lamina lucida, and localized to the proximal part of the anchoring filaments.

PATHOGENESIS

The IgG antibodies are directed against the same antigens as in bullous pemphigoid (BP), i.e. BP180 and BP230. The extracellular region of BP180 adjacent to the transmembrane portion is the immunodominant epitope. In the dermis there is a lymphoyctic infiltrate which has been largely ignored. Whether these lymphocytes are secondary to inflammation of the established lesion is a possibility. However, the lymphocytic infiltrate could represent an early stage in development of the pathological process, resulting in the blister. It has been reported that T cells in PG recognize the same epitope, i.e. the extracellular component of the BP180 antigen[61]. In addition, eosinophils infiltrating the upper dermis are likely to be involved in the pathogenesis of the blister, but probably at a late stage. The chemoattractant factors are yet to be determined. They are possibly related to complement activation or to cytokines released by T cells or keratinocytes.

The antibodies in PG have been shown to be pathogenic in an animal model, as they react with the basement membrane of the amnion placenta and are found in fetal skin and cord blood; they also bind C3 complement, and this binding is easier to demonstrate than the antibodies themselves.

CLINICAL FEATURES

The lesions usually first appear around the umbilicus (Figure 7.2) and then spread over the abdomen and subsequently to the limbs (Figure 7.3), including the

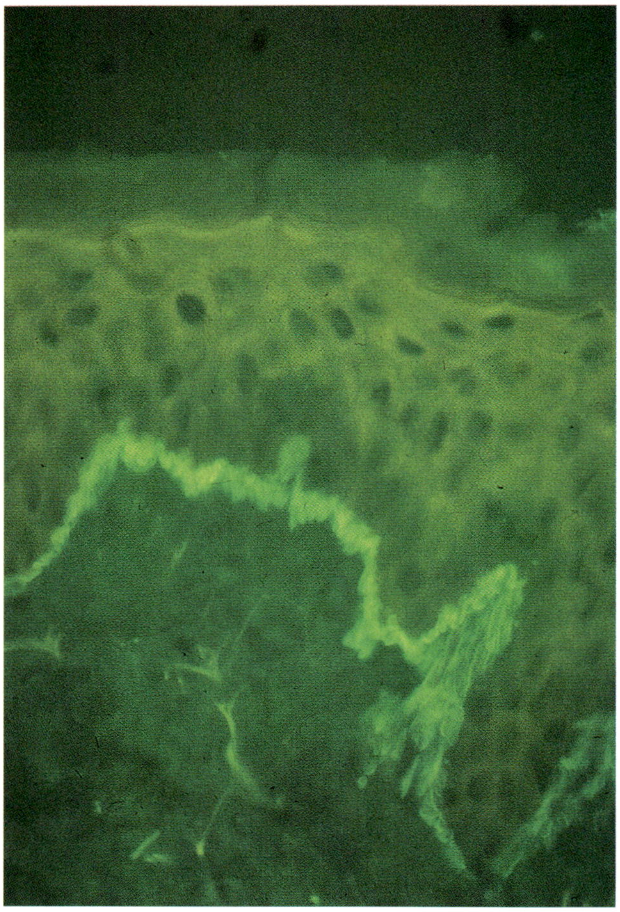

Figure 7.1 Pemphigoid gestationis factor binding C3 to the basement membrane

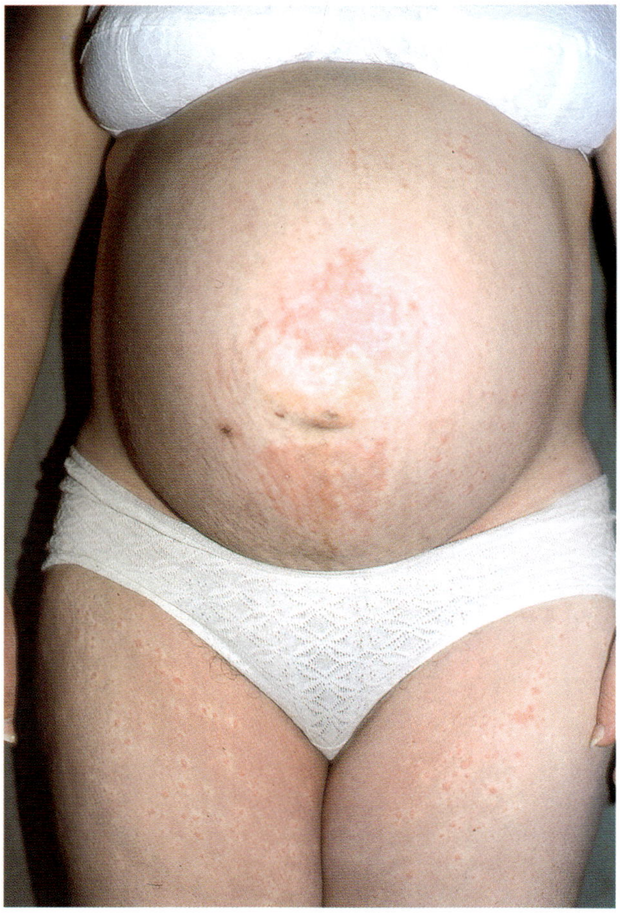

Figure 7.2 Pemphigoid gestationis (PG) usually begins on the abdomen around the umbilicus. The early lesions are erythematous plaques

palms (Figure 7.4) and soles, an uncommon site for other bullous dermatoses. Mucous membrane involvement is uncommon but may occur. The early lesions are urticarial plaques and papules, some with an annular configuration. Blisters then appear on the urticarial lesions. The blisters are of varying size, from 0.5 to 2 cm. PG is intensely irritating.

The eruption may present at any time after the first month of pregnancy, but is most common in the second and third trimesters. In addition, PG may appear for the first time during the first month postpartum.

PG presents in a first pregnancy in approximately 50% of patients. Occurrence in subsequent pregnancies is common, and usually begins earlier than in the previous one. Occasionally PG becomes less severe towards the end of the pregnancy, but may flare postpartum.

TREATMENT

If the disorder is mild, potent topical steroids may help in controlling the eruption. Oral antihistamines may help with irritation. Generally, first-line systemic treatment is with oral corticosteroids, and usually moderate doses, i.e. 20 mg prednisolone daily, are sufficient to control the eruption. Occasionally higher doses are necessary. Successful treatment has also been reported with dapsone. However, hemolysis will occur, and if severe then this drug should be discontinued. Intravenous immunoglobulin has been reported to be successful in some patients, and should be tried if the eruption is not controlled with a moderate dose of corticosteroids. Tetracyclines have been reported to be effective but are contraindicated in pregnancy, but can be used postpartum if the mother is not breast-feeding.

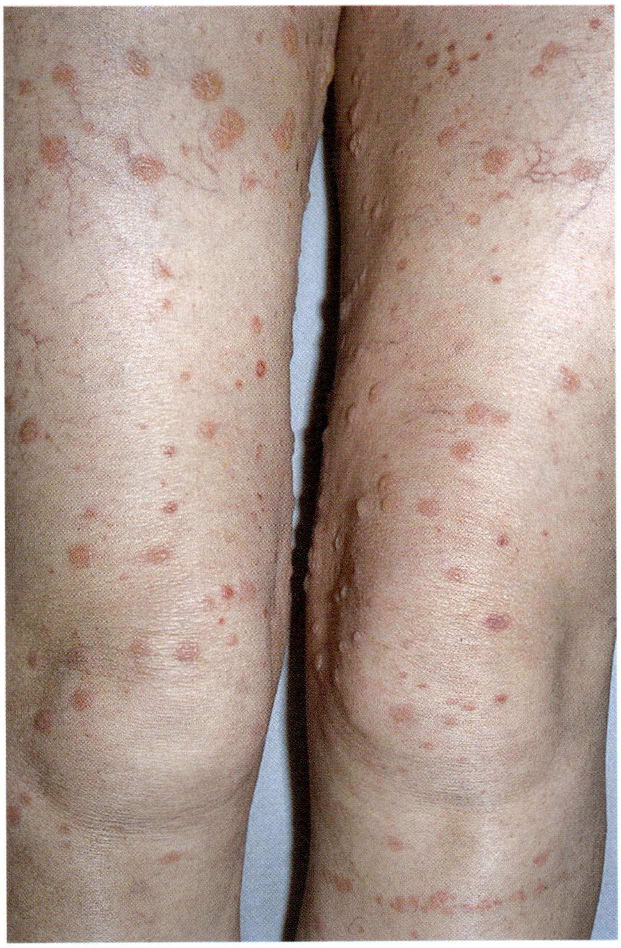

Figure 7.3 Urticarial papules and blisters on the thighs

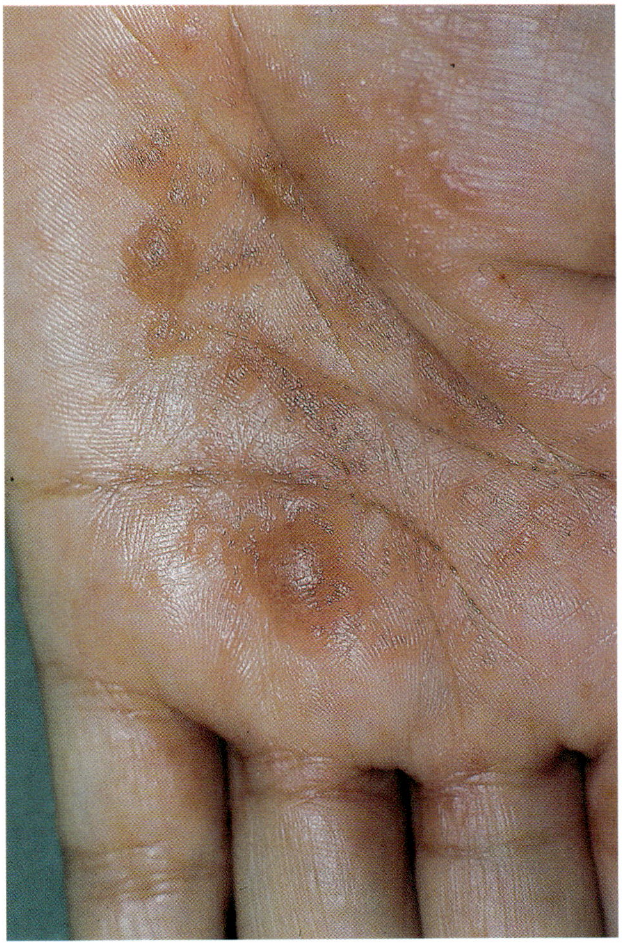

Figure 7.4 Blisters on the palm in PG, an uncommon site for other immunobullous disorders

PROGNOSIS AND NATURAL HISTORY

PG usually clears postpartum, although flares may occur in this period. Very occasionally PG may persist for months and even years. It has been argued that those with persistent disease really have bullous pemphigoid.

PG will usually occur in subsequent pregnancies. In some instances the eruption occurs more early in the subsequent pregnancies and it may also be more severe.

Following PG there may be flares associated with menstruation, but these settle in time.

Since one of the initiating factors is the mismatch of fetal antigens derived from the father and those of the mother, the effect of a different partner in subsequent pregnancies may influence the development of the rash. There are reports of a change of partner lessening the risk of PG, but also reports indicating no effect. It is likely that whether there is a beneficial effect depends on the compatibility between the paternal and maternal antigens.

PG appears to be associated with premature delivery and low birth weight. This is probably due to the effect of the antibodies on the placenta.

ASSOCIATED DISEASES

Not surprisingly as the B8/DR3/DR4 is present in the majority of patients with PG, autoimmune disorders have an increased incidence. Those disorders associated with PG are thyroid disease, vitiligo and alopecia areata.

DIFFERENTIAL DIAGNOSIS

The commonest disorders to be distinguished from PG are the other pregnancy eruptions. Papular eruption of pregnancy usually appears early in pregnancy and may clear before the end of the pregnancy. The papules are usually less than 5 mm and are found mainly on the trunk. No blisters occur, and direct immunofluorescent tests are negative.

Polymorphic eruption of pregnancy is more common than PG, the incidence being 1 : 250 pregnancies. As in PG the eruption usually begins on the abdomen, in striae if present, and spreads to the upper limbs. There is severe irritation, and as the name implies the lesions may be of varied morphology, including urticarial papules and plaques, small blisters and target lesions. The distinction from PG is made by a biopsy from uninvolved skin, in which immunofluorescent studies for C3 and IgG are negative and there is an absence of the 'PG factor' in the serum.

Other disorders associated with severe pruritus but not related directly to pregnancy which also have to be considered are atopic eczema and scabies. The former may be exacerbated by pregnancy.

8 Mucous membrane pemphigoid

Mucous membrane pemphigoid (MMP) is sometimes referred to as cicatricial pemphigoid because it may be associated with scarring. There is an overlap with linear immunoglobulin A (IgA) disease which may also be associated with scarring of the conjunctiva. Not all the ectodermally derived mucous membranes are affected. The eye or the mouth may be affected without the other.

EPIDEMIOLOGY

MMP is a rare disease. In Caucasians the incidence is said to be one per million per year. It appears to be less common in Asians. In a 2-year study of autoimmune subepidermal bullous disorders in Singapore, 67 patients were identified but none had MMP[48]. Similarly, in a study from Kuwait over an 11.5-year period, in which 128 patients with autoimmune bullous disoders were identified, none had MMP[49]. It is possible that patients with mainly or only eye symptoms will present to an ophthalmological center and those with mainly oral lesions will present to oral physicians. Thus, the true incidence may be higher, as patients may present in three different clinics. It has been estimated that the incidence of ocular disease alone is 1 : 1 000 000/year, which is the same as given for Europeans for all manifestations of MMP. MMP is the commonest autoimmune bullous disorder presenting with conjunctivitis.

ETIOLOGY

MMP is classified as an autoimmune bullous disease with antibodies directed against a number of antigens in the basement membrane region. Those described are against the hemidesmosome (BP180, BP230), the anchoring filaments in the lamina lucida and the anchoring fibrils in the dermis (Figure 4.1). As with the other autoimmune bullous disorders, the trigger for the development of antibodies to these antigens is not known. It is possible that an environmental factor, e.g. micro-organisms, may act as a trigger, the alternative being a break in the immunosuppressive function of the immune system, which is another of the possibilities for autoimmune diseases in general.

Human leukocyte antigen (HLA) associations have been reported for MMP. An increase in the allele DQB1*0301 and a decrease in DQB1*02 have been found. The DQB1*0301 encodes a negative charge at position DQ57 (Asp), a critical position for peptide binding to the HLA-DQ molecule, and this may play a part in the selection of peptides[62].

PATHOLOGY

The characteristic feature is a subepidermal blister, but because of the sites of pathology, i.e. oral mucosa and eyes, the blisters rupture easily giving rise to an erosion. There is a lymphohistiocytic infiltrate below the basement membrane. Fibrosis, the characteristic feature of MMP, occurs at a later stage.

As stated above several antigens have been mentioned in MMP. They are the bullous pemphigoid (BP) antigens, BP230, BP180, $\alpha 6\beta 4$ integrin, laminin 5 and collagen VII in the anchoring fibrils. The cause of the scarring is yet to be determined, but is unlikely to be simply the fact that the upper dermis is involved in the pathology. In dermatitis herpetiformis the site of pathology is the upper dermis, but scarring is not a feature of the disease.

Direct immunofluorescence of the perilesional skin and oral mucous membrane shows deposition of C3 and IgG, and less frequently IgA and IgM, along the line of the basement membrane. Biopsy of the conjunctiva is usually positive for the immunoglobulin deposits in only about 50% of patients (Figure 8.1). This may reflect the fact that if the disease is active then, in effect, the biopsies are being taken from involved tissue and not uninvolved, as can be identified for skin and/or mucous membrane biopsies.

Indirect immunofluorescence is positive in about half the patients, and the antibodies may be IgG, IgA or IgM, and there is some correlation with the class of immunoglobulin found on direct immunfluorescence[63].

Immunoelectron microscopic studies show that immunoglobulin deposits are mainly localized to the lamina lucida and lamina densa. This suggests that the antigens are different from those in bullous pemphigoid, and raises the possibility that antibodies to BP180 and BP230 are of a secondary nature.

PATHOGENESIS

The main differences between BP and MMP are: there is a predilection for mucous membrane sites, and scarring occurs, in MMP. The cause for these differences is not known. There are a number of possible explanations. First, the HLA association of MMP (see above) may have an effect on the immunological response in MMP. Second, immunoelectron microscopy studies have shown deposits in the lamina lucida and lamina densa in MMP, but in the hemidesmosome region and lamina lucida in BP. The possibility exists that the primary antigens in MMP are different, being the anchoring fibrils in MMP, whilst in BP they are BP230 and BP180. The fact that antibodies to BP230 and BP180 are also found in the serum in MMP may imply that these antibodies are secondary, resulting from damage in the basement membrane region.

The scarring which is seen in MMP suggests that the primary site of pathology involves the dermis in some way. Damage to the anchoring fibrils may initiate a scarring process, or the pathogenetic pathway involved also results in scarring as well as inducing damage to this region.

Studies of cytokines of the conjunctival tissue have shown a Thl (T helper cell) response, in the inflammatory response, as interleukin-2 (IL-2) and γ-interferon are present[64]. There is an increase in activated T cells, and antigen-presenting cells (dendritic cells and macrophages). These findings raise the possibility that MMP is a T cell-mediated disease, and the binding of antibody to antigen is not the initiating factor in producing the pathology.

Other cytokines found in ocular MMP include fibroblast growth factor (FGF), platelet derived growth factor (PDGF) and transforming growth factor-β (TGF-β)[64]. These cytokines are involved in regulating the extracellular matrix components and fibroblast activity with the production of collagen. The cytokines are produced by inflammatory cells, macrophages and fibroblasts themselves, and may be involved in the scarring process.

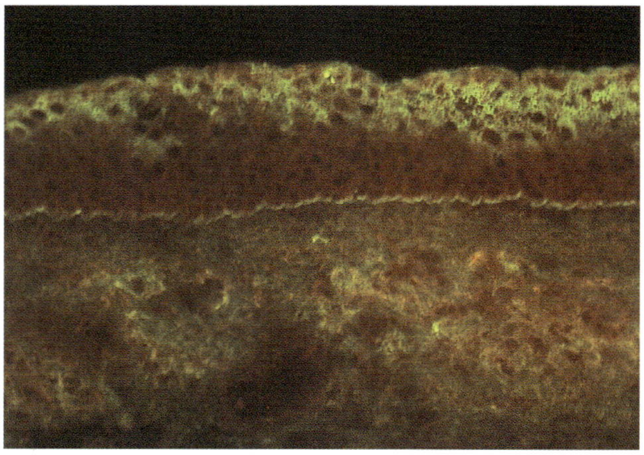

Figure 8.1 Conjunctival biopsy showing immunoglobulin A (IgA) deposits along the line of the basement membrane

CLINICAL FEATURES

MMP is more common in females, with a ratio of 3 : 1. It most commonly presents in the sixth and seventh decades. However, it has also been known to begin in the third, fourth, fifth, eighth and ninth decades.

The clinical features vary according to the site of involvement, and are discussed separately. The sites of involvement are the oral cavity, the pharynx and larynx, the eye, the genitalia and the skin. All of these sites may be involved in a single patient, or only one site, or there may be a combination of two or three sites.

The eye

Initial symptoms include soreness and redness of the eye. Dry eye and mucus deficiency may follow. In a small proportion of patients the disease may be rapidly progressive, with severe inflammation and conjunctival ulceration. If the disease progresses slowly there is subepithelial fibrosis due to increased collagen formation and inflammation. This presents as entropion, shortening of the fornices and symbleph-aron (Figures 8.2 and 8.3). The end stage is fusion of the lids (Figure 8.4) and corneal surface failure (Figure 8.5), leading to blindness. However, the disease is not always progressive, and may become inactive, spontaneously, at any stage.

Oral cavity

There are a number of presentations. Small blisters (Figure 8.6) and erosions (Figure 8.7) may be the presenting features. The erosions are slow to heal and painful, and the commonest sites are the buccal mucosae (Figure 8.8) and palate (Figure 8.6). Desquamating gingivitis (red eroded gums) (Figure 8.9) is another presentation, and is very persistent. Patients tend to complain of bleeding gums when brushing their teeth. Scarring, presenting as adhesions, may occur in established disease. These may be seen between the buccal mucosae and aleveolar process and around the uvula and tonsillar fossae. Involvement of the pharynx and upper esophagus

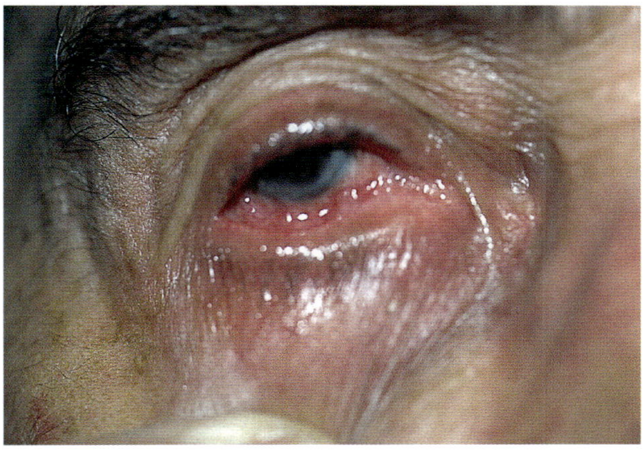

Figure 8.2 Inflamed eye with loss of the lower fornix (the groove between the tarsal and bulbar conjunctiva) and symblepharon (tethering of the bulbar conjunctiva to that of the lower lid)

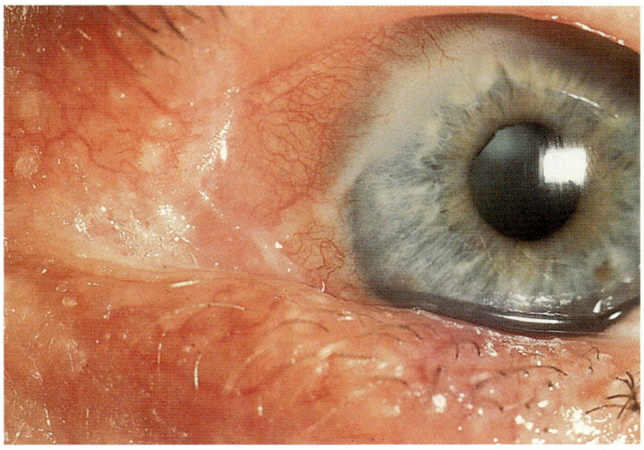

Figure 8.4 Late-stage disease: fusion of upper and lower eyelids

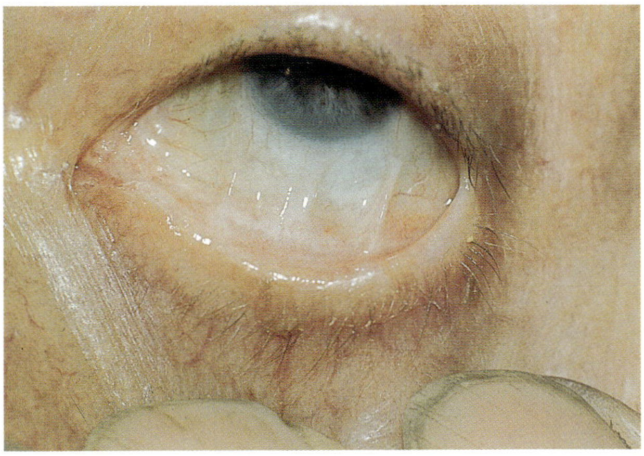

Figure 8.3 Symblepharon in inactive disease: no inflammation present

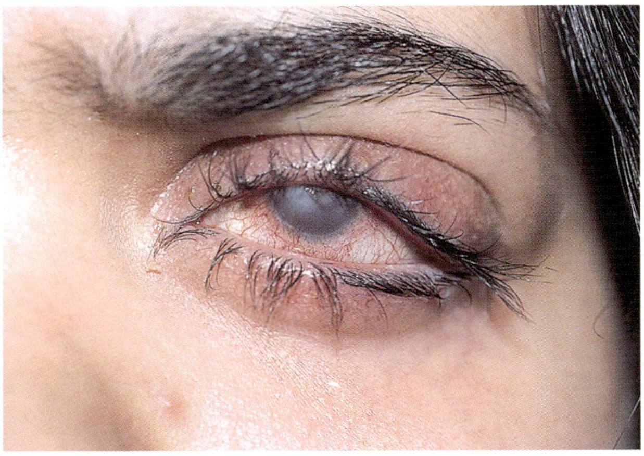

Figure 8.5 Opaque eye with keratinization of the conjunctiva over the cornea

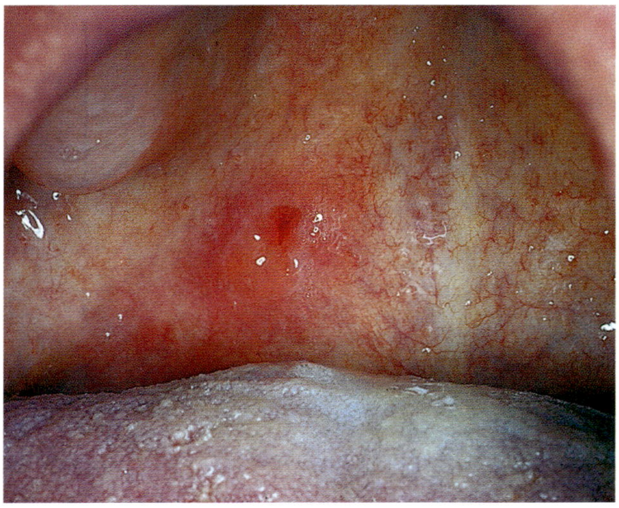

Figure 8.6 Blisters and small erosion on the palate in mucous membrane pemphigoid (MMP)

may progress to stricture formation and present as dysphagia. Involvement of the larynx presents as hoarseness, and if strictures develop asphyxia may occur.

Genital involvement in females presents with blisters and ulceration of the vulva. Introital narrowing may result from scarring, and in the end stage there is labial fusion. In the male, blisters and erosions of the penis occur, and scarring between the glans and foreskin.

The skin lesions occur in approximately 20% of patients, and may be a generalized bullous eruption similar to bullous pemphigoid or they may be few and localized (Figure 8.10). The latter are most common near the orifices and on the scalp (Figure 8.11). They tend to be persistent, with eventual scarring (Figure 8.10).

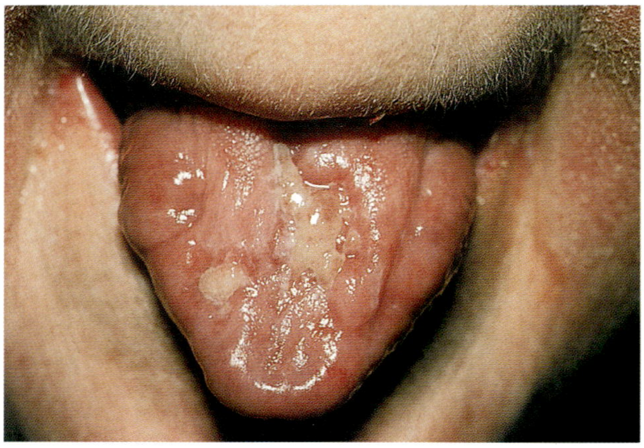

Figure 8.7 Erosions and blisters on the tongue in MMP

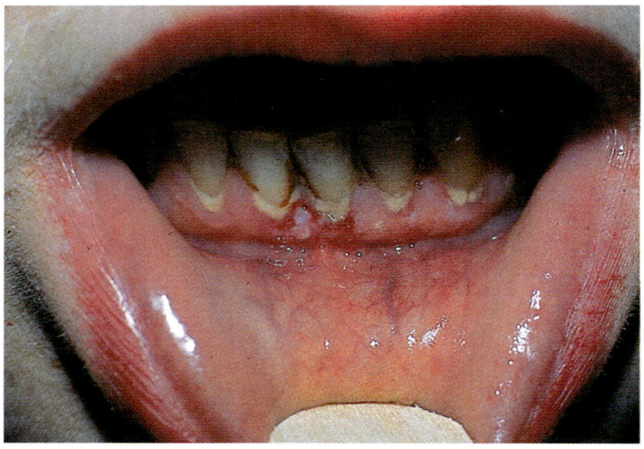

Figure 8.9 Desquamative gingivitis

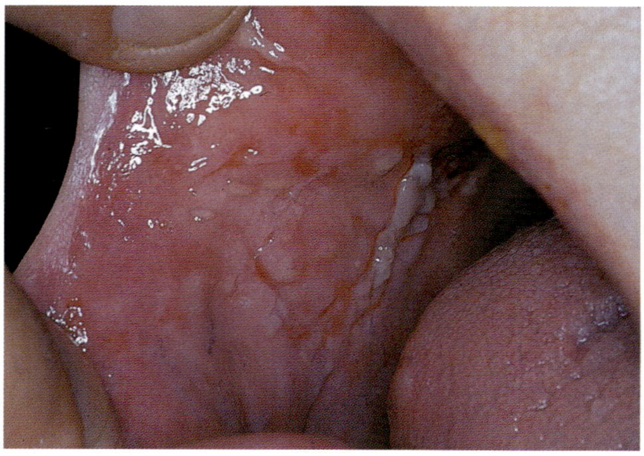

Figure 8.8 Erosions on buccal mucosa

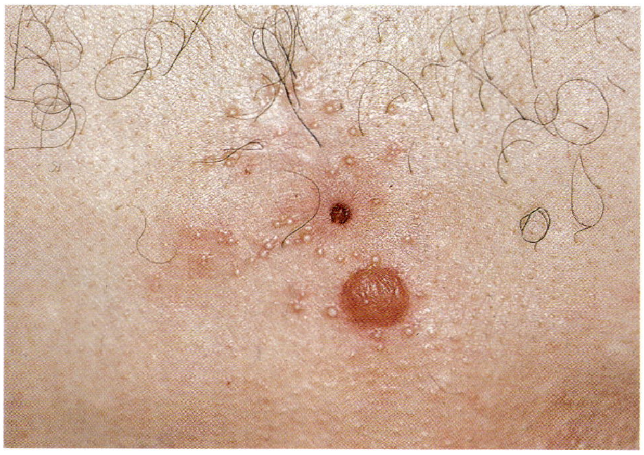

Figure 8.10 Blisters with some scarring in a localized area in MMP

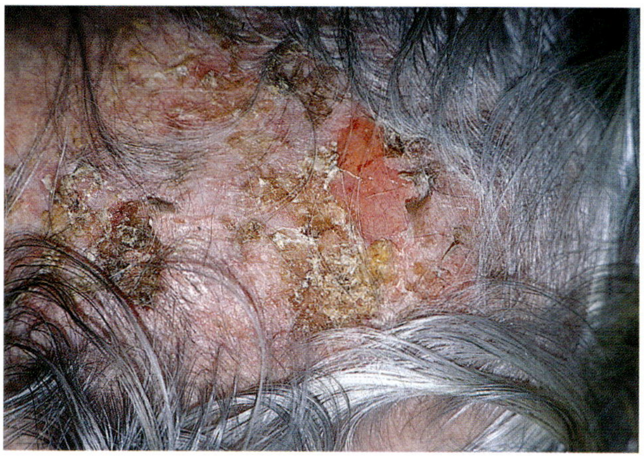

Figure 8.11 Crusting and erosions with hair loss from the scalp in MMP

INVESTIGATIONS

Direct immunfluorescent tests of perilesional skin and/or mucous membranes is the most important investigation. Biopsy of the conjunctiva can be performed by an ophthalmologist; however, the test is not always positive, for the reasons discussed above. Indirect immunofluorescence is positive in only approximately 50% of patients.

TREATMENT

Topical

Although the cutaneous, oral and genital lesions can be managed by a dermatologist, the eye involvement should be jointly or solely managed by an ophthalmologist. Local treatments may be used as the sole medicament or in combination with systemic ones. Potent or very potent steroids may be effective for genital and skin lesions. They may also be helpful for oral lesions when given as a mouthwash or used as a spray (usually from a steroid inhaler for asthma). Tetracycline mouthwashes may also be tried if the steroid ones are not effective.

Systemic treatments

Initial treatment with dapsone or sulfonamides (sulfapyridine or sulfamethoxypyridazine) should be tried, as they are often effective and relatively safe compared with the other drugs used.

Systemic steroids have been used, and are helpful in controlling oral and skin lesions, but they do not appear to be helpful in controlling eye involvement.

Immunosuppressive drugs including azathioprine and cyclophosphamide have been used, the latter particularly for acute ocular flare-ups. There are reports of a favorable response to tetracycline, and this may be given as the sole agent for a trial period or combined with other modalities. Intravenous immunoglobulin has been used with some success.

NATURAL HISTORY AND PROGNOSIS

MMP runs a variable course. In the majority of patients it runs a slow chronic course over many years, and permanent remissions occur in some patients. In the more severe and active disease, depending on which site is involved, there may be blindness, laryngeal and esophageal stenosis, and vulval obliteration with micturition problems. Treatment may abort the progression of the disease but has to be considered as long-term. Some of the treatments themselves carry high morbidity and may even produce fatalities.

DIFFERENTIAL DIAGNOSIS

This depends on the site involved.

The eye

The conditions which have to be distinguished from MMP are severe infections, chronic allergic conditions, erythema multiforme (Stevens–Johnson syndrome), toxic epidermal necrolysis, reactions to topical medicaments and pemphigus, which may also affect the eye and oral mucosa.

Oral cavity

The other causes of desquamative gingivitis include pemphigus and lichen planus. Pemphigus and Behçet's syndrome may present with persistent oral lesions. Linear IgA disease may be associated with persistent mouth ulcers. Immunofluorescent studies of uninvolved tissue and biopsies of the involved sites for routine histology may be necessary to diagnose lichen planus.

Genitalia

In the acute stages when erosions and blisters are present, herpes simplex and other bullous disorders have to be considered, including pemphigus, bullous pemphigoid and linear IgA disease. Behçet's syndrome and recurrent erythema multiforme also have to be considered. Fixed drug eruption is common on male genitalia, as is recurrent herpes simplex. In the late stages, when scarring occurs, lichen sclerosis is the most likely differential diagnosis.

Skin lesions

If there is a generalized bullous eruption then bullous pemphigoid and linear IgA disease have to be considered. Localized disease on the scalp with scarring may be produced by discoid lupus erythematosus or lichen planus. Fixed drug eruption or dermatitis artefacta can produce persistent lesions with eventual scarring.

9 Epidermolysis bullosa acquisita

Epidermolysis bullosa acquisita (EBA) is a rare disorder. It is so named because of its similar appearance to genetic dystrophic epidermolysis bullosa.

EPIDEMIOLOGY

EBA is probably the rarest of the acquired immunobullous disorders seen in Caucasians, with an incidence of 0.25 per million per year. It appears to be more common in Blacks and Asians. In a report from Singapore of a study of 67 patients with subepidermal bullous diseases, four (6%) had EBA[48]. Although bullous pemphigoid was by far the commonest, with an incidence of 88%, EBA was the second commonest. In a study from Kuwait of 128 patients, all with autoimmune bullous disorders, the incidence was 2.3%, giving an estimated incidence of 0.23 per million per year[49].

ETIOLOGY

The environmental factor which produces the skin lesions is trauma. Thus, the lesions tend to arise at sites of chronic trauma, e.g. the elbows, and the dorsa of the hands and feet. There was a human leukocyte antigen (HLA) association with DR2 in the USA[65], but this was not found in a study from Korea[66]. This discrepancy of HLA antigens in different ethnic groups is not uncommon in immunological disorders.

PATHOLOGY

The blister is subepidermal. In the early stages there is little cellular infiltrate, but in the later stages there is heavy neutrophilic infiltration. Immunofluorescent studies show a linear band of immunoglobulin G (IgG) and C3 complement along the line of the basement membrane. Split-skin studies show that the deposits are on the dermal side of the blister (Figure 1.2). IgA and IgM may also be seen in some patients. Indirect immunofluorescent studies reveal circulating antibodies in approximately half the patients. Immunoelectron microscopy shows immunoglobulin deposits to be located in the upper dermis below the lamina densa.

PATHOGENESIS

Collagen VII of the anchoring fibrils in the upper dermis is the target antigen in EBA. Collagen VII comprises non-collagenous components and a collagenous component. The antibodies in EBA are directed against the non-collagenous component.

There is some evidence that the autoantibodies are pathogenic[67] and bind complement, which is responsible for the attraction of neutrophils into the skin. Probably, enzymes released from the activated neutrophils induce the damage to the tissue with resultant blister formation.

CLINICAL FEATURES

EBA may occur in any age group, including children. There is no sex predilection reported.

The commonest areas to be involved are at the sites of trauma, i.e. the dorsa of the hands and feet (Figures 9.1 and 9.2) and the elbows. Blisters develop, and the surrounding skin is red and scaly. Scarring will eventually occur. Milia are a common

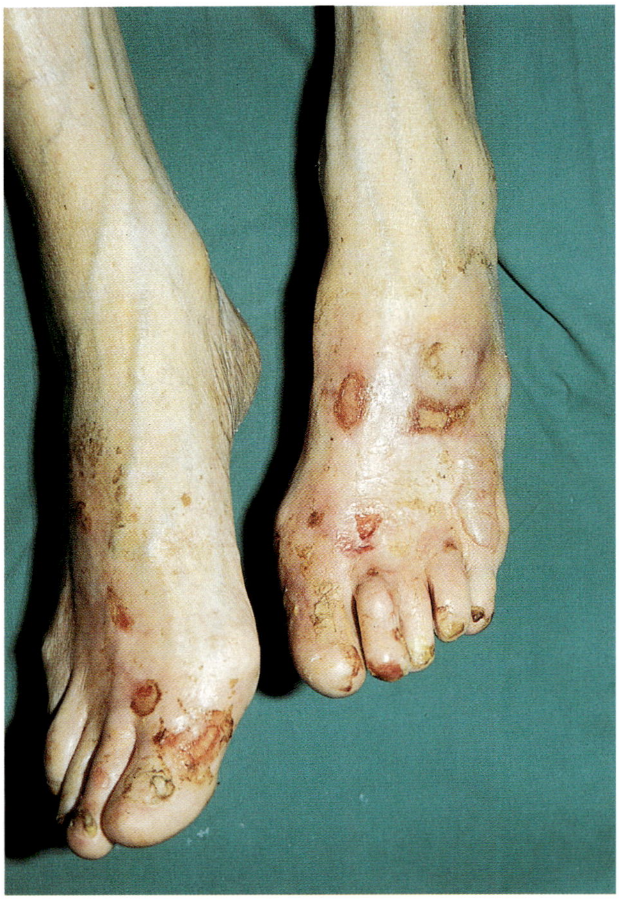

Figure 9.1 Bilateral epidermolysis bullosa acquisita (EBA): erosions on dorsa of the feet, a common site

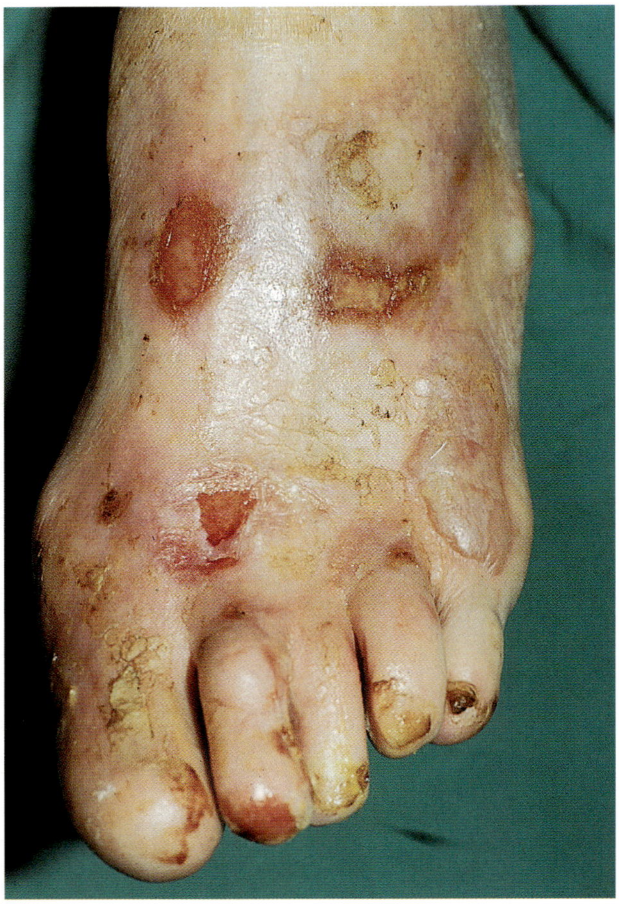

Figure 9.2 Blisters and erosions on dorsum of the foot. Some scarring is present

feature in the healed skin. Nails may become dystrophic if the nail matrix is involved.

Another form of presentation is a widespread bullous eruption (Figure 9.3), as seen in linear IgA disease or bullous pemphigoid.

Involvement of the mucous membranes may occur, with erosions and blisters. The sites of involvement are the mouth, pharynx, larynx and the upper esophagus. EBA is included as one of the causes of cicatrizing conjunctivitis.

TREATMENT

Dapsone and sulfonamides (sulfapyridine and sulfamethoxypyridazine) are sometimes effective, probably by inhibiting the migration and activation of the neutrophils. Systemic corticosteroids and the immunosuppressive agents azathioprine and cyclosporine have also been used, and are claimed to be helpful. Intravenous immunoglobulin has also been tried with some success. As EBA is so rare in the Western world, there are very few large detailed studies of the most effective treatment.

PROGNOSIS AND NATURAL HISTORY

EBA limited to the sites of trauma tends to be persistent. However, remissions have been reported in patients with widespread disease. Long-term treatment will be necessary for the localized forms of the disease. Scarring and loss of nails may interfere with functions of the hands and feet.

DIFFERENTIAL DIAGNOSIS

When EBA is localized to sites of trauma, particularly in young persons, it has to be distinguished from the inherited form of dominant epidermolysis bullosa. The distinction can be made by positive direct immunofluorescence and lack of family history in EBA. Mucous membrane pemphigoid (MMP) produces similar mucous membrane lesions and scarring, but does not usually involve the hands and feet. Immunofluorescence may help to distinguish the two conditions if the immunoglobulin deposits are in the roof of the blister, using split skin as the substrate in MMP. However, the deposits may be in the floor of the blister, as in EBA.

Porphyria cutanea tarda produces blisters and scarring on the back of the hands. However, other exposed areas such as the face are not usually involved in EBA. In addition, porphyrin studies and immunofluorescent studies will distinguish between the two conditions. If EBA presents as a widespread bullous eruption it will have to be distinguished from bullous pemphigoid and linear IgA disease (LAD). Immunofluorescent studies using the split-skin technique will distinguish EBA from bullous pemphigoid, as in the latter the deposits are in the roof of the blister. The distinction from LAD is made by the class of immunoglobulin, although IgG as well as IgA may be found in LAD and deposits may also be found in the floor of the blister.

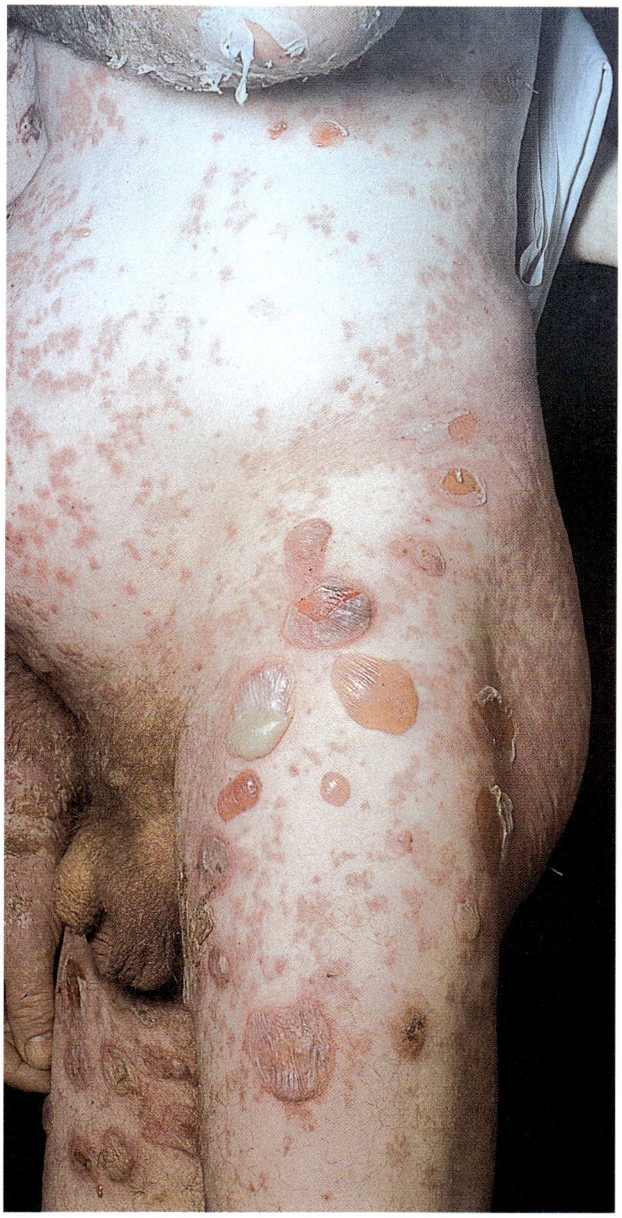

Figure 9.3 Widespread bullous eruption which may occur in EBA

10 Mixed bullous disease

AN ENTITY?

It has been argued that the subepidermal blistering diseases may represent a spectrum of disease and not clearly defined entities. This overlap may occur in the clinical features, immunoglobulin class, site and pattern of immunoglobulin deposition and so-called target antigens (Table 10.1).

CLINICAL

Although there are characteristic sites for the eruption in a number of the disorders, for example the extensor regions of elbows and knees and the buttocks in dermatitis herpetiformis (DH), periumbilical region in pemphigoid gestationis (PG) and pubic region in childhood linear immunoglobulin A (IgA)

Table 10.1 Overlap of clinical and immunological features of subepidermal bullous disorders

	Urticarial plaques with blisters	*Mucous membrane involvement*	*Immunoglobulin class*	*Pattern of deposition*	*Site*	*Antigen(s)*
BP	+	(+)	IgG (IgA)	Linear	Epidermal	BP180 BP230
LAD	+	+	IgA (IgG)	Linear	Epidermal	BP180 BP230
					Dermal	collagen VII
PG	+	(+)	IgG	Linear	Epidermal	BP180 BP230
MMP	–	+	IgG, IgA	Linear	Epidermal	BP180 BP230
					Dermal	$\alpha6\beta4$ integrin laminin 5 collagen VII
EBA	+	(+)	IgG	Linear	Dermal	collagen VII
DH	+	(+)	IgA (IgG)	Granular (linear granular)	Dermal	reticulin tissue-transglutaminase

BP, bullous pemphigoid; LAD, linear IgA disease; PG, pemphigoid gestationis; MMP, mucous membrane pemphigoid; EBA, epidermolysis bullosa acquisita; DH, dermatitis herpetiformis; +, major feature; (+), minor feature; (Ig), class of immunoglobulin found occasionally disease, difficulty in making a diagnosis will arise if the eruption is widespread, as may occur with any of them. The age of onset may be a pointer to the correct diagnosis, for example childhood linear IgA (LAD), young adults in DH and the elderly in bullous pemphigoid (BP), but there is considerable overlap between these disorders. DH may commence in the elderly and BP in young or middle-aged adults.

Morphology of the lesions may be similar in many of the subepidermal bullous disorders. One of the commonest is blisters arising on urticarial plaques, which can be present in DH, BP, PG, LAD and epidermolysis bullosa acquisita (EBA). Tense blisters may occur in all these disorders. However, if scarring of the skin is present, then this will limit the diagnosis to either mucous membrane pemphigoid (MMP) or EBA.

Although mucous membrane involvement is common in MMP and LAD, it may also occur in all the other subepidermal bullous disorders. However, it is usually severe only in MMP and LAD.

SITE AND PATTERN OF IMMUNOGLOBULIN DEPOSITION

Direct immunofluorescence of the uninvolved skin has now become the most reliable test for establishing the diagnosis. This test, if positive, will tend to exclude the non-autoimmune bullous diseases and the epidermal from the subepidermal types. However, in all the subepidermal disorders, except DH, the pattern of deposition is linear along the line of the basement membrane. Even in DH, in approximately 10% of patients a linear pattern of IgA along the line of the basement membrane is present. However, this linear band is not homogeneous as in the other subepidermal bullous disorders. The linear band in DH has breaks in it and is referred to as 'linear granular'.

If the 'split-skin test' is used, it is possible to increase the sensitivity of the test. Immunoglobulin deposition in the roof of the blister is seen in BP, MMP, PG and LAD, and on the floor of the blister in EBA and DH. However, deposition on the floor of the blister may also be seen in MMP and LAD, and rarely in BP. Thus, deposition of immunoglobulin may occur at two sites in the same subepidermal disease entity. The two different sites of deposition imply that there are different antigens in these 'entities', which may in fact represent two different disorders.

The class of immunoglobulin deposition may help in establishing the correct diagnosis. It is commonly IgG in BP, PG, MMP and EBA, whilst it is IgA in LAD and DH. However, IgG may also occur in DH and LAD, but this is in addition to IgA, which is always present. IgA can also be found in MMP, either in addition to IgG or as the sole class of immunoglobulin. Thus, some overlap, whether it is the class or pattern of immunoglobulin deposition, occurs in this group of disorders.

THE ANTIGENS

A number of target antigens have been postulated over the past two or three decades in the group of subepidermal disorders, and some are common to them. BP180 and BP230, the postulated antigens of BP, have also been found to be present in MMP, PG and LAD. Collagen VII, a constituent of the anchoring fibrils, has been reported to be one of the antigens in LAD, MMP and EBA. The finding that antigens may be common to a number of bullous disorders raises two important points. First, there is overlap between the subepidermal bullous disorders, and these antigens are not specific to any one entity. Second, the antibodies that are used to define these antigens may be secondary antibodies from damage to the skin induced by some other factor, possibly of an environmental nature.

The exception to a common antigen in the subepidermal bullous disorders is DH. The autoantigen in DH and celiac disease has now been defined as tissue-transglutaminase. However, the induction of antibodies to tissue-transglutaminase is due to an external factor, namely gluten, and the antibodies disappear with gluten withdrawal.

HUMAN LEUKOCYTE ANTIGENS

The haplotype Al/B8/DR3 is increased in DH, LAD and PG. This haplotype is also found in other non-dermatological autoimmune disorders, and there is an increase of these disorders in DH, PG and LAD. Thus, there is a common genetic basis for a number of these subepidermal bullous disorders.

RESPONSE TO TREATMENT

Before the advent of detecting immunogloubilin deposits in the skin, one of the criteria for diagnosing DH was the response of the rash to dapsone. However, it has now been seen that this is not a reliable test for making a diagnosis. All the other subepidermal bullous disorders show varying degrees of improvement with dapsone. In addition, there are other non-bullous skin disorders which respond to dapsone. Dapsone appears to influence the trafficking and activation of neutrophils in the skin, and thus acts on a common pathway at the end-stage of a pathogenetic mechanism in blister formation in bullous diseases.

CONCLUSION

Thus, although the subepidermal bullous disorders have been divided into a number of entities, there is considerable overlap in their clinical, immunological and etiological features and response to treatment. Further study in the future may determine whether the current terms for the subepidermal bullous disorders reflect distinct entities or a spectrum of disorders with overlapping features.

11 Subcorneal bullous dermatosis

Subcorneal bullous dermatosis (SCBD) is a relatively rare dermatosis characterized by a flaccid blister and the accumulation of neutrophils in the subcorneal region of the epidermis.

PATHOLOGY

In the early stages there is a dermal perivascular infiltrate mainly of neutrophils and eosinophils. The neutrophils migrate up through the epidermis to the subcorneal region where they collect to form a fluid-filled blister. Immunofluorescent studies are negative, although there are occasional reports of immunoglobulin A (IgA) in the intercellular space of the epidermis.

PATHOGENESIS

The pathogenesis is poorly understood. The chemoattractant factors for the neutrophils have not been investigated, although interleukin-8 (IL-8) has been shown to be present in the stratum corneum and granular region of the epidermis. If IL-8 were the chemoattractant, it is not known what up-regulates its production.

There are reports of SCBD being associated with an IgA monoclonal gammopathy[68] and pyoderma gangrenosum[68,69], which is also associated with neutrophil infiltration. Although in some patients intercellular IgA has been found, it is possible that this is a variant of IgA pemphigus and not SCBD.

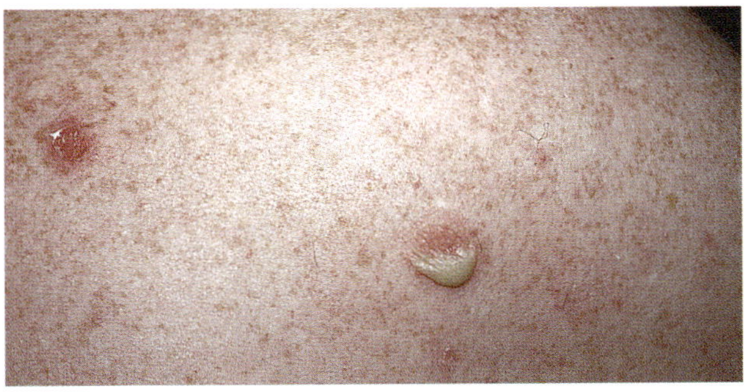

Figure 11.1 Flaccid blister with neutrophils in the lower half of the blister. Also present is a crusted lesion, on the medial back, which is due to a ruptured blister

CLINICAL FEATURES

SCBD is commoner in females and usually presents in middle-aged adults. The main lesion is a flaccid blister with pus cells in the lower half of the lesion (Figure 11.1). These cells will move as the patient changes position, e.g. from lying to standing. The blisters tend to arise from normal skin (Figure 11.1), rupture easily and give rise to a superficial crusted area (Figure 11.1). The lesions often appear in crops, suggesting that a central factor is determining their initiation. However, sometimes they present as individual blisters.

The lesions occur mainly on the limbs; the trunk may be affected but the face and scalp are usually not involved.

NATURAL HISTORY AND PROGNOSIS

SCBD tends to be a persistent disorder, although eventual remission occurs after a number of years.

TREATMENT

The eruption responds well to dapsone and the sulfonamides, sulfapyridine and sulfamethoxypyridazine. Often, smaller doses than that required for dermatitis herpetiformis are effective. Dapsone is thought to influence the migration of neutrophils. Once control of the eruption has been obtained, the dose of the drug should be gradually decreased to see whether a remission has occurred.

Other treatments that have been claimed to be effective include colchicine and ultraviolet light (both narrow-band UVB and PUVA (psoralen and UVA)).

DIFFERENTIAL DIAGNOSIS

The commonest differential diagnosis is impetigo. This can usually be determined by taking a swab for bacteriology.

Prior to immunofluorescent studies, SCBD was often diagnosed as dermatitis herpetiformis because the eruption responded to dapsone.

If IgA is present in the intercellular space of the epidermis, then it is likely that the correct diagnosis is so-called IgA pemphigus, which also responds to dapsone.

Generalized pustular psoriasis presents with sheets of pustules which are usually smaller and more numerous. In addition, in pustular psoriasis the onset is sudden, and may be accompanied by constitutional upset. There is usually also a history of plaque psoriasis.

References

1. Gawkrodger DJ, Blackwell JN, Gilmore HM, et al. Dermatitis herpetiformis: diagnosis, diet and demography. Gut 1984; 25: 151–7
2. Reunala T, Lokki J. Dermatitis herpetiformis in Finland. Acta Derm Venereol 1978; 58: 505–10
3. Christensen DB, Hindsen M, Svensson A. Natural history of dermatitis in Southern Sweden. Dermatologica 1986; 173: 271–7
4. Fry L. Dermatitis herpetiformis. In Howdle PD, ed. Clinical Gastroenterology: Coeliac Disease. London: Bailliere Tindall, 1995: 371–94
5. Wong SN, Chua SH. Spectrum of subepidermal immunobullous disease seen at the National Skin Centre, Singapore: a 2 year review. Br J Dermatol 2002; 147: 476–80
6. Shibahara M, Nanko H, Shimizu M, et al. Dermatitis herpetiformis in Japan. An update. Dermatology 2002; 202: 37–42
7. Reunala T. The incidence of familial dermatitis herpetiformis. Br J Dermatol 1996; 134: 394–8
8. Hervonen K, Hakanen M, Kaukinen K, et al. First degree relatives are frequently affected in celiac disease and dermatitis herpetiformis. Scand J Gastroenterol 2002; 37: 51–5
9. Hervonen K, Kasell K, Holopainen P, et al. Concordance of dermatitis herpetiformis and coeliac disease in monozygotic twins. J Invest Dermatol 2000; 115: 990–3
10. Jepson LV, Ullman S. Dermatitis herpetiformis and gluten sensitive enteropathy in monozygotic twins. Acta Derm Venereol 1980; 60: 353–5
11. Kosnai I, Karpati S, Torok B. Dermatatis herpetiformis in monozygous twins: discordant for dermatitis herpetiformis and concordance for gluten sensitive enteropathy. Br J Paediatr 1985; 144: 404–5
12. Spurkland A, Ingvarsson O, Falk ES, et al. Dermatitis herpetiformis and coeliac disease are both primarily associated with HLA-DQ (alpha 1*0501, beta 1*02) or the HLA-DQ (alpha 1*03, beta 1*0302) heterodimers. Tissue Antigens 1997; 49: 29–34
13. Balas A, Vicario L, Zambrano A, et al. Absolute linkage of coeliac disease and dermatitis herpetiformis to HLA-DQ. Tissue Antigens 1997; 50: 52–6
14. Greco L, Romino R, Coto I, et al. The first large population based twin study of coeliac disease. Gut 2002; 50: 624–28
15. Holopainen P, Mustalhti K, Umara P, et al. Candidate gene regions and genetic heterogeneity in gluten sensitivity. Gut 2001; 48: 696–701
16. Houlston RS, Tomlinson IP, Ford D, et al. Linkage analysis of candidate gene regions for coeliac disease genes. Hum Med Genet 1998; 62: 1335–9
17. Greco L, Babron MC, Coraza GR, et al. Existence of a genetic risk factor on chromosome 5q in Italian coeliac families. Am Hum Genet 2001; 65: 35–41
18. Diosdado B, Wapenaar MC, Franke L, et al. A microarray screen for novel candidate genes in coeliac disease pathogenesis. Gut 2004; 53: 944–51
19. Fry L, McMinn RM, Cowan JD, Hoffbrand AV. Effect of a gluten-free diet on dermatological, intestinal and haematological changes in dermatitis herpetiformis. Lancet 1968; 1: 557–61

20. Seah PP, Fry L, Hoffbrand AV, Holbarrow EJ. Tissue antibodies in dermatitis herpetiformis. Lancet 1971; 2: 834–6

21. Unsworth DJ, Johnson GD, Haffenden G, et al. Binding of wheat gliadin in vitro to reticulin in normal and dermatitis herpetiformis skin. J Invest Dermatol 1981; 76: 88–93

22. Dietrich W, Bhnis T, Bauer M, et al. Identification of tissue transglutaminase as the autoantigen in coeliac disease. Nat Med 1997; 3: 797–801

23. Sardy M, Karpati S, Merkl B, et al. Epidermal transglutaminase (TGase3) is the autoantigen in dermatitis herpetiformis. J Exp Med 2002; 10: 747–57

24. Eckert RL, Sturniolo M, Broome A-M, et al. Transglutaminase function in epidermis. J Invest Dermatol 2005; 124: 481–92

25. Ermarcora E, Prampolini L, Tribbja G, et al. Long term follow-up of dermatitis herpetiformis in children. J Am Acad Dermatol 1986; 15: 24–30

26. Wojnarowska F, Fry L. Hepatic injury in dermatitis herpetiformis. Acta Derm Venereol 1981; 61: 165–8

27. Alexander JO'D. Dermatitis Herpetiformis. London: WB Saunders, 175

28. Garioch JJ, Lewis HM, Sargent SA, et al. 25 years experience of a gluten-free diet in the treatment of dermatitis herpetiformis. Br J Dermatol 1994; 131: 541–5

29. Leonard JN, Haffenden GP, Tucker W, et al. Gluten challenge in dermatitis herpetiformis. N Engl J Med 1983; 308: 816–19

30. Lewis HM, Reunala T, Garioch JJ, et al. Protective effect of gluten-free diet against development of lymphoma in dermatitis herpetiformis. Br J Dermatol 1996; 133: 363–7

31. McFadden JP, Leonard JN, Powles AU, Fry L. Autoimmunity in dermatitis herpetiformis: effect of a gluten-free diet. J Dermatol Treat 1991; 2: 87–9

32. Toscano V, Conti FG, Anastasi E, et al. Importance of gluten in the induction of endocrine autoantibodies in adolescent celiac disease. Am J Gastroenterol 2000; 95: 1742–8

33. Hummel M, Bonifacio E, Naserke HE, Ziegler AG. Elimination of dietary gluten does not reduce titers of type 1 diabetes-associated autoantibodies in high-risk subject. Diabetes Care 2002; 25: 1240–1

34. Freeman HJ. Lymphoproliferative and intestinal malignancies in 214 patients with biopsy defined coeliac disease. J Clin Gastroenterol 2004; 38: 429–34

35. Hervonen K, Vornanen H, Kautianen H, et al. Lymphoma in patients with dermatitis herpetiformis and their first degree relatives. Br J Dermatol 2005; 152: 82–6

36. Holmes GKT, Prior P, Lane MR, et al. Malignancy in coeliac disease – effect of a gluten-free diet. Gut 1989; 30: 333–8

37. Korman NJ. Pemphigus. Dermatol Clin 1990; 8: 689–700

38. Aboobaker J, Morar N, Rarndul PK, Hammond MG. Pemphigus in South Africa. Int J Dermatol 2001; 40: 115–19

39. Ahmed AR, Yunis EJ, Khatri K, et al. Major histocompatibility complex haplotype studies in Ashkenazi Jewish patients with pemphigus vulgaris. Proc Natl Acad Sci USA 1990; 87: 7658–62

40. Loiseau P, Lecleach L, Prost C, et al. HLA class II polymorphism contributes to specific desmoglein-derived peptides in pemphigus vulgaris and pemphigus foliaceus. J Autoimmun 2000; 14: 67–71

41. Moraes JR, Moraes ME, Fernandez-Vina M, et al. HLA antigens and risk for development of pemphigus foliaceus (fogo selvagem) in endemic areas of Brazil. Immunogenetics 1991; 33: 388–91

42. Bystryn J-C, Rudolph JL. Pemphigus. Lancet 2005; 366: 61–73

43. Arin M, Engert A, Kreig T, Hunzelmann N. Anti-CD20 monoclonal antibody (rituximab) in the treatment of pemphigus. Br J Dermatol 2005; 153: 620–5

44. Kamradt T, Goggel R, Erb KJ. Induction, exacerbation and inhibition of allergic and autoimmune disease by infection. Trends Immunol 2005; 26: 259–67

45. Bernard P, Vaillant L, Labeille B, et al. Incidence and distribution of subepidermal autoimmune bullous skin disease in three French regions. Arch Dermatol 1995; 131: 48–52

46. Zillikens D, Wever S, Roth A, et al. Incidence of autoimmune subepidermal blistering dermatoses in a region of central Germany. Arch Dermatol 1995; 131: 956–8

47. Gudi VS, White MI, Cruickshank M, et al. Annual incidence and mortality of bullous pemphigoid in the Grampian region of North-east Scotland. Br J Dermatol 2005; 152: 424–7

48. Wong SN, Chua, SH. Spectrum of subepidermal immunobullous disorders seen at the National Skin Centre, Singapore: a 2 year review. Br J Dermatol 2002; 147: 476–80

49. Nanda A, Dvorak K, Al-Saeed K, et al. Spectrum of autoimmune bullous disease in Kuwait. Int J Dermatol 2004; 43: 876–81

50. Banfield C, Wojnarowska F, Allen J, et al. The association of HLA-DQ7 and bullous pemphigoid is restricted to men. Br J Dermatol 1998; 138: 1085–90

51. Liu Z. Are anti-BP180 IgGI or IgG4 antibodies pathogenic? J Invest Dermatol 2002; 119: 989–90

52. Jin P, Shao C, Ye G. Chronic bullous dermatosis in China. Int J Dermatol 1993; 32: 89–92

53. Wojnarowska F, Marsden A, Bhogal B, et al. Chronic bullous disease of childhood, childhood cicatricial pemphigoid and linear IgA disease of adults: a comparative study demonstrating clinical and immunpathological overlap. J Am Acad Dermatol 1988; 19: 792–805

54. Kelly S, Frith P, Millard P, et al. A clinical pathological study of mucosal involvement in linear IgA disease. Br J Dermatol 1988; 119: 161–70

55. Cooper SM, Powell J, Wojnarowska F. Linear IgA disease successful treatment with erythromycin. Clin Exp Dermatol 2002; 27: 677–9

56. Burge S, Wojnarowska F, Marsden A. Chronic bullous dermatosis of childhood persisting into adulthood. Paediatr Dermatol 1988; 5: 246–9

57. Paige D, Leonard J, Wojnarowska F, et al. Linear IgA disease and ulcerative colitis. Br J Dermatol 1997; 136: 779–82

58. Godfrey K, Wojnarowska F, Leonard J. Linear IgA disease of adults with lymphoproliferative malignancy and possible role of other triggering factors. Br J Dermatol 1990; 123: 447–52

59. Kolodny RC. Herpes gestationis. A new assessment of incidence, diagnosis and fetal prognosis. Am J Obstet Gynecol 1969; 104: 39–45

60. Shornick JK, Bangert JL, Freeman RG, et al. Herpes gestationis: clinical and histological features of 28 cases. J Am Acad Dermatol 1983; 8: 214–24

61. Lin MS, Gharnia MA, Swartz S, et al. Identification and characterisation of epitopes recognised by T lymphocytes and autoantibodies from patients with herpes gestationis. J Immunol 1999; 162: 4991–7

62. Drouet M, Delpuget-Bertin N, Vaillent L, et al. HLA-DRB1 and HLA-DQBl genes in susceptibility and resistance to cicatricial pemphigoid in French Caucasians. Eur J Dermatol 1998; 8: 330–3

63. Leonard JN, Hobday CM, Haffenden GP, et al. Immunofluorescence studies in ocular cicatricial pemphigoid. Br J Dermatol 1988; 118: 209–17

64. Elder MJ, Dar JK, Lightman S. Conjunctival fibrosis in occular cicatricial pemphigoid – the role of cytokines. Exp Eye Res 1997; 65: 165–76

65. Gammon W, Hesse E, Burke W, et al. Increased frequency of HLA-DR2 in patients with auto-antibodies to epidermolysis bullosa acquisita antigen; evidence that expression of autoimmunity to type VII collagen is HLA class II allele associated. J Invest Dermatol 1988; 91: 228–32

66. Lee CW, Kim SC, Han H. Distribution of HLA class II alleles in Korean patients with epidermolysis bullosa acquisita. Dermatology1996; 193: 328–9

67. Woodley DT, Chang C, Ram SP, et al. Evidence that antitype VII collagen antibodies are pathogenic and responsible for the clinical, histological and immunological features of epidermolysis bullosa acquisita. J Invest Dermatol 2005; 125: 958–64

68. Carter H, Plantin P, Leroy JP, et al. Pyoderma gangrenosum, subcorneal IgA pustulosis and recurrent neutrophilic pleural and pulmonary diseases in a patient with IgA gammopathy. Ann Derm Venereol 1993; 122: 97–101

69. Delporte E, Colombel JF, Nguyen-Mailfer C, et al. Subcorneal pustular dermatosis in a patient with Crohn's disease. Acta Derm Venereol 1992; 72: 301–2

Index